Supreme Health and Fitness by Sean Ali !

PRESENTS:

UNDERSTANDING

CARBOHYDRATES:

LIFE Energy,

Fiber,

Sugar

and Starch!!

Science Of Life Series ..... Volume 3

Supreme Health and Fitness by Sean Ali!

Achieving and Maintaining Supreme Health and Fitness by increasing the level of Knowledge and Science of Life!

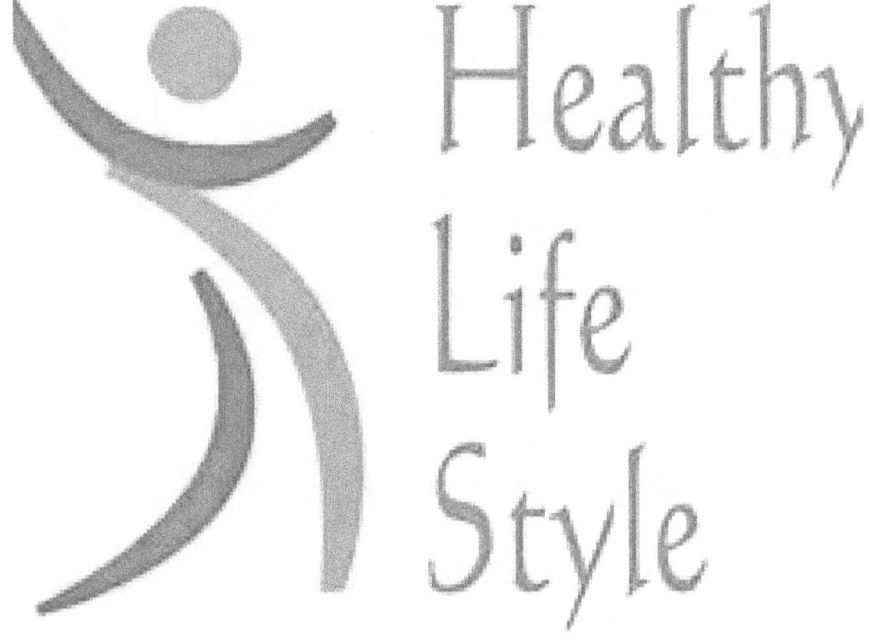

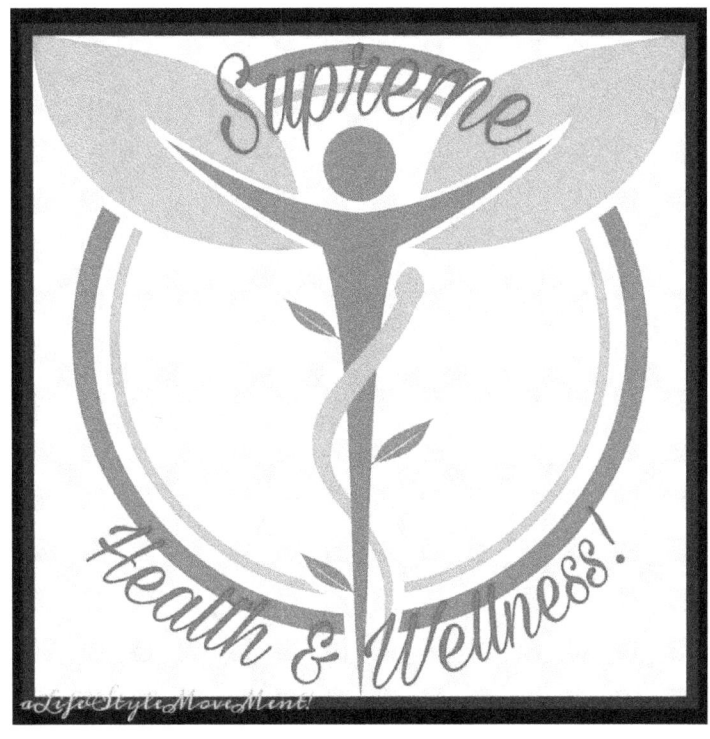

Dedicated to the LifeStyle MoveMent of Growing Our Own Food!

Assisting Scientists:

*Khalil Malik * Kareem Tyree * Gabriella Monique*

Table of Contents

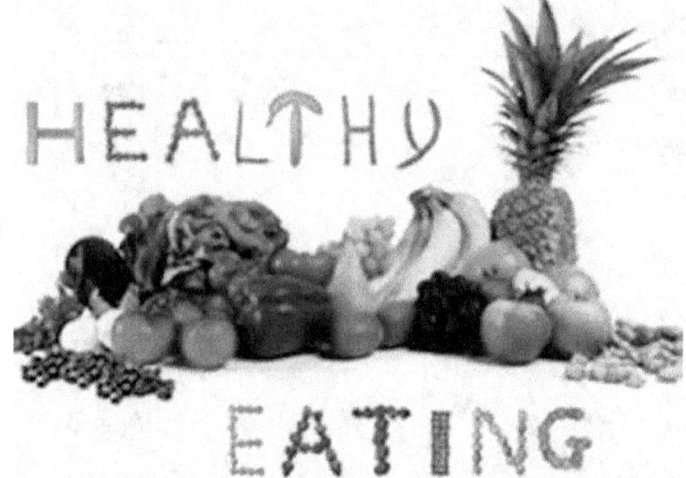

Introduction

* * * * *

Carbohydrates are the most Essential and Integral element in our diet and lives which has been almost unchanged over the course of time as well as nurturing various cultures throughout the world as the major source of Energy for work and growth. Recently researchers, dieticians and food manufacturers have focused attention on Digestible and Indigestible Carbohydrates and how they individually and collectively present various effects on our health. One main elements of Carbohydrates is manifested in the form of an Indigestible Carb, commonly referred to as Fiber and has specific functions in maintaining gastrointestinal health which is the foundation of TOTAL Body Health and Wellness.

There are several natural Plant foods that have been identified as Functional Foods (Life Foods) that have Natural properties that positively Promote and Influence health.

Unfortunately, added Sugars that are processed and manufactured and which contribute KCalories but NO Nutritional value, are making up a greater proportion of the typical American, replacing the needed Complex Carbohydrates and Fiber.

There is a disproportionate amount of fad diets and food-like items available that promote a detrimentally 'low' or 'no' Carb meal plan that goes TOTALLY against ALL Nutritional Science and evidence of the function and role of Carbohydrates.

There is very little to no serious regulation of these types of claims made on labels or advertised as health and fitness. Most are cases of clever advertisement vs actual claims of quality and value.

This small book has been produced to provide the Nutritional and Life value of Carbohydrates from a Scientific analogy with the secondary intent of shedding light on the false and health damaging un-scientific claims.

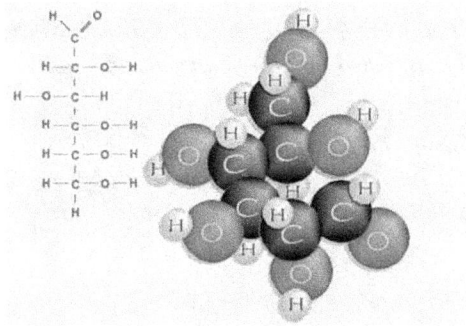

Understanding Carbohydrates: Life Energy, Fiber, Sugar & Starch!

In order for us to achieve our maximum Physical potential, we have to begin to look at ourselves and Nutrition from the Natural Scientific perspective with an understanding that our Nutrition is ONLY found in Nature.

We come from the Earth and ALL our SOLUTIONS come from the Earth ...All we have to do is turn back to the Earth and Extract what we need. We extract what we need by Harvesting from the Bountiful supply of naturally occurring Fruits and Veggies.

The Sun is the sole source of LIFE Energy for Any and All Biological systems of Life in the Universe. Nutrition, whether in the form of Micro-Nutrients = Vitamins and Minerals or Macro-Nutrients = Carbohydrates, Lipids or Protein, are simply different manifestations and expressions of the Energy of the SUN.

WE ARE PEOPLE OF THE SUN !!

We receive the LIFE Energy from the Sun through one of 2 ways = ABSORBING (Sun-bathing) and DIGESTION (Eating).

We Absorb the LIFE Energy of the Sun through the Synergistic relationship between the Sun and the Atoms of our SKIN. Standing in the Sun and Sun-Bathing is an actual Medical Prescription and the 1ˢᵗ way we 'ate'.

Energy cannot be destroyed, only transformed and transferred in form.

The vegetation of Earth are the perfected vehicles to take the Unseen LIFE Energy of the Sun and transform it into Seen Chemicals that we can digest to extract the LIFE Energy that we need to live.

Carbohydrates are the BEST Manifestation of the Sun's LIFE Energy in Chemical or Food form for us to digest. The radiant LIFE Energy of the Sun converts the Atoms and Molecules of the plants into these Carbohydrate, forming the Chemical Bonds of the Atoms that form it.

The Nature of the Carbohydrate

Our bodies require a variety of Nutrients, but there are only a few specific Nutrients needed to achieve and maintain Homeostasis as well as the growth, maintenance and repair of our many Cells and Tissues, which is our foundation.

The Nutrients that we need are normally divided into six classes that include: Carbohydrates, Fats, Proteins, Vitamins, Minerals, and Water. With the exception of Water, ALL of these Life Elements are the SEEN properties that are manifested from the UNSEEN Energy of the Sun!

Understanding Carbohydrates: Life Energy, Fiber, Sugar & Starch!

Understanding Carbohydrates, their importance and function in our diet as well as in almost all our bodily functions, we have the ability to make better food choices which in turns manifests in an overall Improvement our Health and Fitness which allows us to lead a full and active Life.

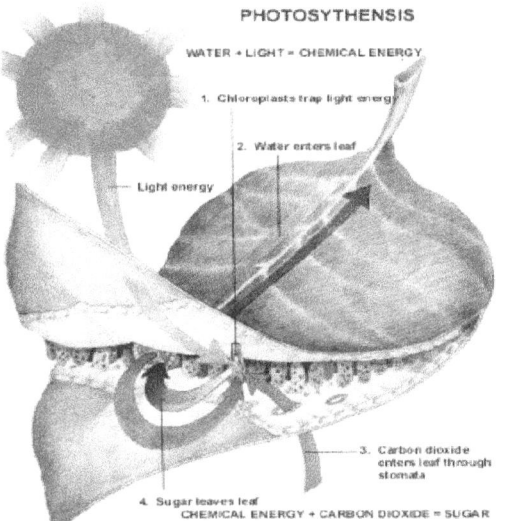

We have a physical Body or Vehicle that is created to literally last Forever. They are finding bones that are being carbon-dated as being well over 2 million years old, so we have a vehicle that's almost indestructible. Now, how we treat this Magnificently Crafted Vehicle determines how long we get to Enjoy it.

How we FEED our Body determines how LONG we have to Reside in it. With a proper Understanding of the Science of Nutrition and that the food we consume as Bio-Fuel also has a simultaneous effect on our Mental and Spiritual bodies, which are the other components which classifies LIFE, we can Successfully Build and Maintain Supreme Health and Fitness = LIFE Abundant !!

Carbohydrates provide as many Mental health benefits for us as they do for our Physical body. Our Central Nervous System is dependent upon the Sun-Light that is manifested as CARBOHYDRATES!

We are either eating to Die or Eating To LIVE ....There is no In-Between !!!!!!

The food choices we make will only serve one of 2 functions = cause Pre-Mature Death......or LIFE Abundant !!

We are People Of The SUN......And Regardless of what any Nutritional Element is called, it is ONLY a by-product of the SUN's LIFE Energy.

Understanding the intricate relationship between ourselves and the SUN will help us Build ourselves to Perfection!

EATING CARBOHYDRATES IS EATING THE SUN !!!!

Achieving and Maintaining Supreme Health and Fitness by increasing the level of Knowledge and quality of the Sciences of LIFE!

PEACE

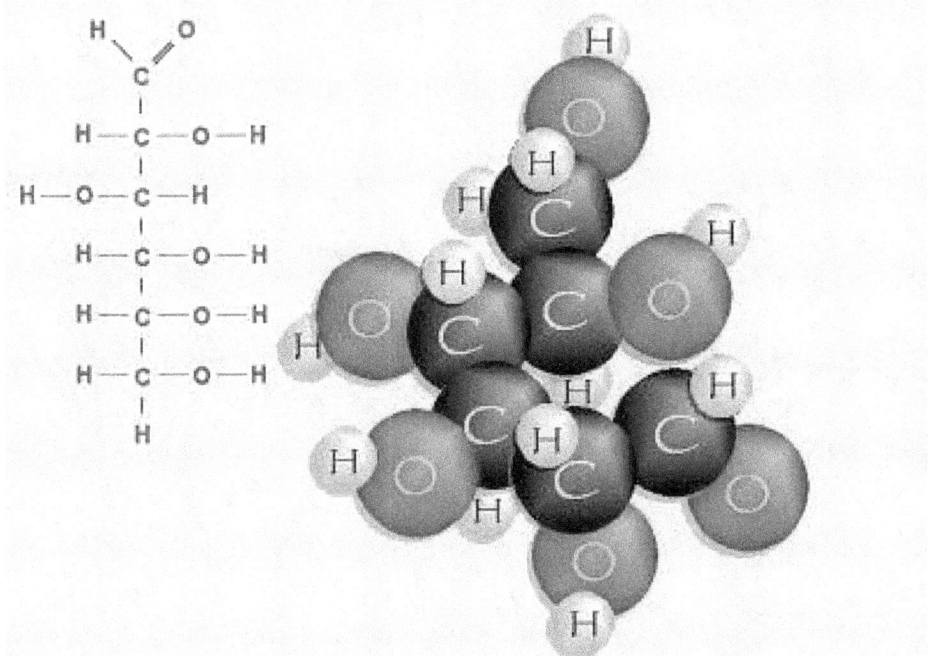

Chapter 1: Importance of Carbohydrates

* * * * *

The Complex Carbohydrate found in Vegetables, Legumes, and Grains must be considered and treated as the Major Dietary Source of Energy.

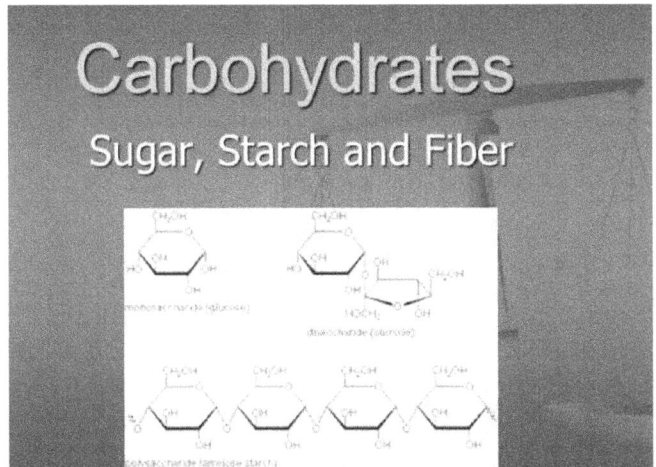

Our bodies are products of the Earth, the same elements and chemical composition.

Our Health and Life Energy is supplied from the Elements of the Earth, manifested in the form of the foods that we consume.

We just have to simply turn back to the Earth and extract the Nutrients that we need.

Our Life-Energy manifests in the form of CARBOHYDRATES.

During Digestion, Starch manifests Glucose, which is the favorite and preferred Energy source of the Body and more specifically our Cells. Fruit and Dairy products supply Carbohydrates in the form of naturally occurring Sugars - Fruit contains Fructose, and Milk contains Lactose.

Vegetables, Legumes, Fruits, and Grains (especially Whole Grains) supply other important Nutrients, including Vitamins, Minerals, and Fiber.

Whole Milk and the dairy products created from present good sources for our supply of natural Calcium, Magnesium, and Protein.

Currently, the major food-like sources of Starch in the American diet are Refined Grains, such as white bread, white sugar and ready-to-eat cereals, white potatoes, pasta, and rice, which are often highly processed and severely limited in Micronutrients and may manifest more detrimental qualities versus any Nutritional value

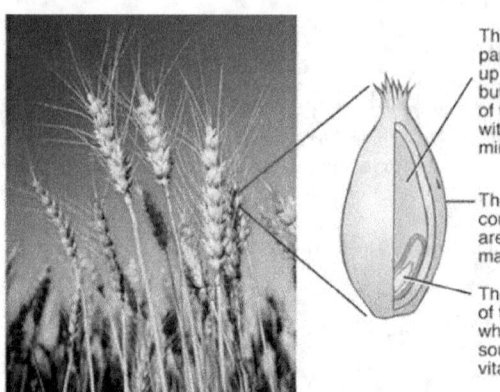

THE THREE UNHEALTHY WHITES

WHITE RICE   WHITE FLOUR   WHITE SUGAR

When you eat a bowl of oatmeal or a slice of whole-wheat toast, you are consuming a Whole-Grain product. Whole-Grain products include the entire Kernel of the Grain: the Germ, the Bran, and the Endosperm.

In Refined (Un-Natural, Processed and Manufactured) Grain products, such as the Toxic white bread, include just the Endosperm and the functionally valuable Bran and nutritionally valuable Germ are discarded during these refining procedures.

In addition to that, the Fiber, along with some vital Vitamins and Minerals are lost/destroyed, which now renders the final refined/processed product Nutritionally Void and potentially Harmful to our Health.

To make up for some of these losses, the Refined Grains sold in the United States are required to be enriched. Enrichment is a totally Unnatural process which is an attempt to add back some, but not all, of the naturally occurring Nutrients lost in processing.

The difference is that that Nutrients that are destroyed are Naturally Occurring Chemical compositions of the SUN. The Enriching procedure is adding elements that were constructed in a laboratory, completely devoid of the SUN.

The **endosperm** is the largest part of the kernel. It is made up of primarily starch, but it also contains most of the kernel's protein, along with some vitamins and minerals.

The outermost **bran** layers contain most of the fiber and are a good source of many vitamins and minerals.

The **germ**, located at the base of the kernel, is the embryo where sprouting occurs. It is a source of oil and is rich in vitamin E.

An example of the Nutrients destroyed are, the Thiamin, Niacin, Riboflavin, and Iron that are lost when Whole Grains are milled are later added back to levels that are equal to or higher than originally present.

The DANGER is that these companies use man-made versions of these natural elements and these manufactured elements no longer have the LIFE Energy of the SUN through Photosynthesis. So, when our Bodies attempt to Metabolize these unnatural elements, negative unnatural Energy is released, in the form of Free-Radicals, instead of Natural LIFE Energy from the SUN.

Since 1998 the government has mandated that Folic Acid also be added to the Nutritionally DEFICIENT Refund Grains.

Other nutrients, including Vitamin E and Vitamin B6 are also removed by milling, but they are not added back. Therefore, foods made with these refined grains contain more of some nutrients and less of others than foods made from whole grains.

****REFINED IS THE CATCHPHRASE FOR NUTRITIONALLY DEFICIENT!!!!****

So, the difference is that Whole Grains include the Nutritionally valuable Germ, or inside of the Kernel as well as the Bran covering of the Grain Kernel when compared with refined grains from which the bran has been removed.

We must remember when in a situation where we are about to consume a food-like product that contains Refined grains, that they are enriched with several unnatural elements of B Vitamins, Iron,

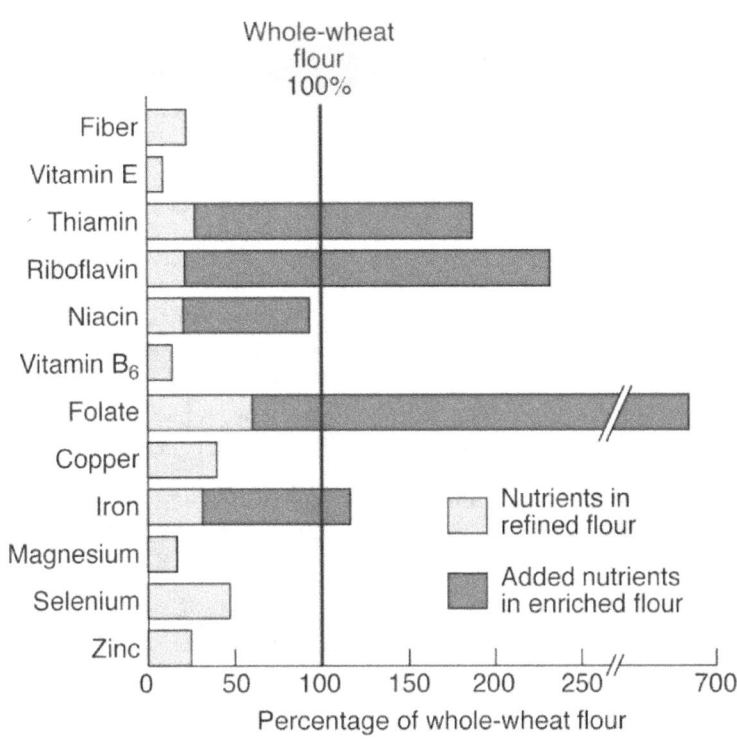

b. The amounts of many nutrients in refined flour (yellow bars) are much lower than the amounts originally present in the whole grain (100% line). In enriched flour, thiamin, riboflavin, niacin, iron, and folate have been added back in amounts that equal or exceed the original levels (red bars).

and Folate that are manufactured and/or processed, but provide less of the needed dietary Fiber and other important trace Minerals.

Refined Carbohydrate rich food-like items that are high in added Sugar offer a supply Kcals but provide little to nothing else in regards to Nutrients. Viewed in conjunction to the research on the connection between added sugar and cardiovascular risk factors, including obesity, the American Heart Association (AHA) recommends a limited intake of these types of Refined Carbs not to exceed 100 kcal per day for women and 150 kcal for men, (AHA, 2016).

Good vs. Bad Carbs

Good	Bad
non-starchy vegetables	soda
starchy vegetables	white pasta
fruits	white rice
greens	sugary cereal

fibrous fruits & veggies > white foods (flour, rice, sugar)

Even though it's clearly evident that these Refined Carbs are detrimental to our Health, instead of BANNING them from being manufactured, the government allows the companies to continue to make these Toxic elements and they are allowed to call their products food.

The best manifestation of Carbohydrates presents in the form of the Whole Wheat Grain.

Carbohydrate Recommendations or the RDA for our total Carbohydrate intake is approximately 130 grams a day, which is based on the estimated Average Minimum amount of Glucose used by the Brain. In a diet that meets Energy needs, this amount provides adequate Glucose which allows for maximum Brain function as well as prevents Ketosis. This means that those that are deficient or don't reach their RDA of Carbs are at risk for decrease in Mental capacity and function that has a serious impact on our ability to produce and maintain Thoughts or Thinking.

A diet that's rich in naturally occurring Carbs is required in order to manifest the highest qualities of our Humanity and explore, discover and create any and everything we can conceive. The ability to Say BE and it Becomes.

Most low-income people/families have little to no access to quality unrefined food sources of Carbohydrates and the level of education compared to people/families with better access are stark in comparison with those with adequate access to Carbs out-performing the former.

Ketosis is a metabolic state in which some of the body's Energy supply comes from Ketone bodies in the Blood, in contrast to the natural state of Glycolysis in which Blood Glucose provides most of the Energy

A limited level or supply of Carbs interferes with Fat break-down, which is a health concern because most of the Energy stored in the body is stored as Fat (Potential Energy).

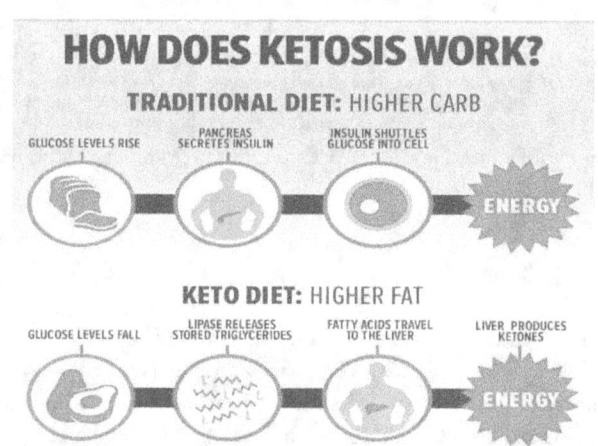

HOW DOES KETOSIS WORK?

TRADITIONAL DIET: HIGHER CARB

GLUCOSE LEVELS RISE — PANCREAS SECRETES INSULIN — INSULIN SHUTTLES GLUCOSE INTO CELL — ENERGY

KETO DIET: HIGHER FAT

GLUCOSE LEVELS FALL — LIPASE RELEASES STORED TRIGLYCERIDES — FATTY ACIDS TRAVEL TO THE LIVER — LIVER PRODUCES KETONES — ENERGY

Understanding Carbohydrates: Life Energy, Fiber, Sugar & Starch!

In our bodies, Fatty Acids are broken down into Two-Carbon Units that forms Acetyl-CoA. In order to continue through Aerobic Metabolism stage, the Acetyl-CoA must combine with a Molecule derived primarily from Carbohydrate. When our Carb supply is deficient then the Acetyl-CoA Molecules cannot continue through the Aerobic Metabolism process and instead they react with each other, combine and form Molecules of Ketones or Ketone bodies.

The Heart, Muscles, and Kidney are able to process and use Ketones for Energy. When undergoing a fast, after about three days even the Brain adapts and can obtain approximately half of its Energy from Ketones. The use of Ketones for energy helps spare Glucose and helps to decrease the amount of Protein that our bodies have to use in order to synthesize Glucose.

Ketone or Ketone Body is an Acidic Molecule formed when there is not enough sufficient Carbohydrates to break down Acetyl-CoA to create LIFE Energy.

Usually the Ketones not used for Energy can be excreted in the Urine. However, when the production of Ketones is high, they build up in the Blood, which is the formation of Ketosis. A mild, but still serious health concern, of Ketosis can occur when consuming a low-carbohydrate weight-loss diet and can cause symptoms such as reduced appetite, headaches, dry mouth, and odd-smelling breath. The condition of excessive Ketones is a direct Effect that is usually Caused by the consumption of Refined, manufactured and/or processed Carbohydrates.

Severe Ketosis can occur with untreated diabetes and can cause a detrimental increase in the Blood's Acidity to the level causes our normal body processes to become disrupted, resulting in coma and even death.

Additional Carbs provide an important source of Energy in our diet, and Carbohydrate-containing foods can add Vitamins, Minerals, Fiber, and Phytochemicals that otherwise wouldn't be available or cannot be obtained from other food sources.

The *Acceptable Macronutrient Distribution Range* for Carbohydrates in our diet is set between a minimum of 45% to 65% of our total Calorie intake and a diet within this range meets Energy needs without contributing excessive amounts of Protein or Fat, which have a level of toxicity if too much of either element exceeds their respective RDAs.

A diet that falls below the minimum percentage of 45% means that they are consuming either more Protein or Fat (or both), to replace the Energy that our Bodies would have processed from our primary source of Carbs. The excessive consumption of these Fats and Protein increases both their percentages beyond their respective RDAs.

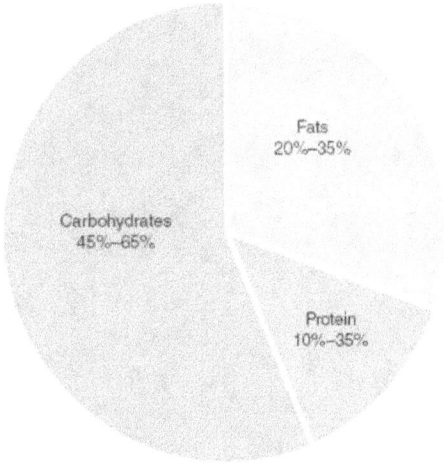

Understanding Carbohydrates: Life Energy, Fiber, Sugar & Starch!

Both Fats and Protein are needed by our bodies to achieve Homeostasis, but we only need limited amounts and excessive Fats and Carbs are a direct Cause that is responsible for the detrimental health Effects of Cardiovascular dis-ease, Diabetes and Obesity.

Because there is no specific toxicity thats associated with high intake of any type of Carbohydrates, no UL has been established for total Carbohydrate intake, for Fiber intake, or for added Sugar intake.

*To *Calculate* the *Percentage* of **KCalories** from **Carbs** in a diet, you first determine the *Number* of **Grams** of **Carbohydrates** and *Multiply* this value by **4** Calories/Gram.

Compare energy sources	
Energy Source	**Calories per gram**
Fats	9
Proteins	4
Carbohydrates	4

For example, using a food that provides about 300 Grams of Carbohydrates:

*300 Grams × 4 KCalories / Grams = 1200 KCalories from Carbohydrates.

*Next *Divide* the number of KCalories from the Carbs by the total number of KCalories in the diet and *Multiply* by 100 to convert it to a *Percentage*. For the example that we are using the diet contains a total of 2000 **KCalories**, which would provide the following:

*(1200 **KCalories** from **Carbs** / 2000 **KCalories** total) × 100 = 60% of **KCalories** from Carbohydrates.

DIETARY FIBER AND ENERGY CONTENT OF SELECTED FOODS

FOOD GROUP	SERVING SIZE	DIETARY FIBER (g)	ENERGY (kcal)
Grains Group			
All Bran (wheat flakes)	¾ cup	5.0	95
Wheaties	¾ cup	2.7	95
Shredded wheat (plain)	2 biscuits	5.5	155
Instant oatmeal, cooked	1 package	4.0	150
Cheerios	1 cup	2.6	106
Air-popped popcorn	1 cup	1.2	31
Whole-wheat bread	1 slice	1.9	81
Vegetable Group			
Kidney beans, canned	½ cup	4.4	99
Green peas, frozen, cooked	½ cup	4.4	62
Corn, frozen, cooked	½ cup	2.0	66
Potato, baked, with skin	1 medium	3.8	161
Carrots, raw	1 medium	1.7	25
Broccoli, chopped, frozen, cooked	½ cup	2.8	26
Spinach, frozen, cooked	1 cup	7.0	65
Fruit Group			
Apple, with skin	1 small	3.6	77
Strawberries, sliced	1 cup	3.3	53
Orange	1 medium	3.1	62
Banana	1 medium	3.1	105

Data from U.S. Department of Agriculture, Agricultural Research Service. 2013. USDA National Nutrient Database for Standard Reference, Release 26. Nutrient Data Laboratory Home Page, http://www.ars.usda.gov/ba/bhnrc/ndl.

Chapter 2: Choosing Carbohydrates Wisely

* * * * *

To promote a healthy, balanced diet we must have an increase in the consumption of Whole Grains, Fruits, Vegetables and Whole Milk, while severely limiting and/or eliminating foods that are high in refined grains and added sugars, which includes ALL soft drinks and other sweetened beverages, sweet bakery products, and candy.

Because the majority of the added sugars Americans consume come from beverages, the Dietary Guidelines specifically recommend severely reducing to completely eliminating our intake of ANY processed/manufactured sugar-sweetened beverages such as soda, energy drinks, sports drinks, and especially sugar-sweetened fruit drinks.

Healthy Fibrous Carbs	Healthy Starchy Carbs	Healthy Simple Carbs
• Vegetables in general. • Cucumbers, asparagus, broccoli, peas, etc. • Squash, carrots, peppers • Tomatoes • Beans	• Grains generally • Whole grains • Whole grain pasta • Beans • Whole grain bread • Potatoes, sweet potatoes • Healthy cereals	• Fruits generally • Apples, orange, bananas, sweet potatoes, pineapple, berries, etc. • Avoid foods with sugar as an ingredient • Avoid most fruit juices, especially non-fresh squeezed

Make half your grains whole

- Have your sandwich on whole-wheat, (oat bran, rye, or pumpernickel bread can be substituted or added but Wheat is the BEST).

- Switch to Whole-Wheat pasta (strive to make your own to avoid the harmful chemicals added to commercial products) and brown rice.

- Instead Of commercial items, fill your cereal bowl with plain oatmeal and add a few raisins for sweetness

> **refined** Refers to foods that have undergone processing that changes or removes various components of the original food.

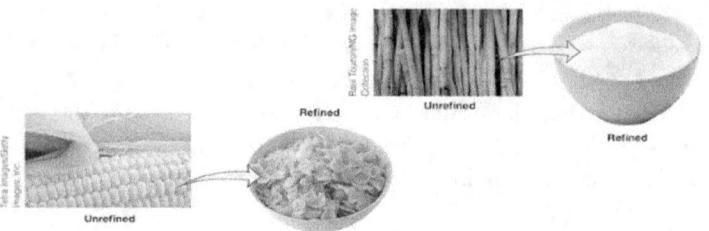

- Check the ingredient list for the words *Whole* or *Whole Grain* BEFORE the grain ingredient's name.

Increase your fruits and veggies

- Don't forget beans. The excellent Navy Bean (other Legumes aren't as digestible or valuable as Navy Beans) has more Fiber and Resistant-Starch than any other vegetables.

- Add naturally sweet and delicious Berries and other Fruit as healthy versions of dessert or snack if you have one.

- Pile the Veggies on your sandwich.

- Have more than one vegetable at dinner or EAT ALL Veggies !!!!!

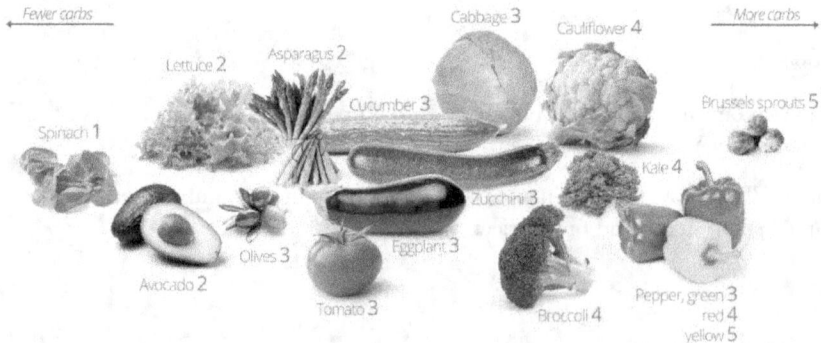

Limit added sugars

- Switch to a 12-oz can instead of a 20-oz bottle IF you grab a soft drink OR, better yet, have a glass of Water or Whole Milk.

- Use only Natural formed Sugars or sweetness like Honey in your recipe to replace artificial ones.

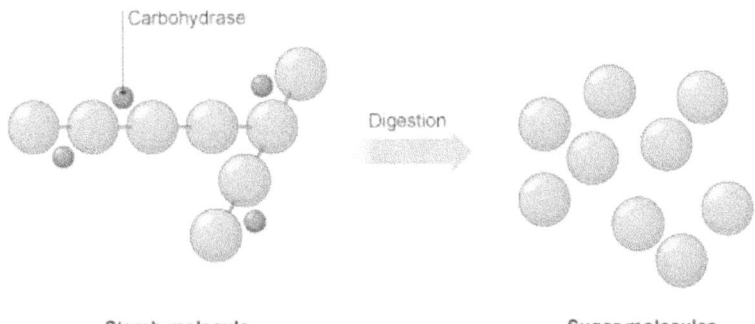

Starch molecule   Sugar molecules

- Snack on a piece of Fruit INSTEAD of a candy bar.

- SWAP your sugary breakfast cereal for an unsweetened Whole-Grain variety.

Chapter 3: Functions of Carbohydrates

* * * * *

The Primary function of Carbohydrates is to be the Chemical Composition of the Un-Seen Power of ththe SUN as a Natural way to supply this LIFE Energy to our Cells, especially those in our Control Center = Brain Cells, which Glucose is vital to. When Carbs are lacking, Fats are our back-up and can be used as a secondary Energy source by most of our Organ and Systems, but this way is limited because our Body Cells and Tissues require a constant supply of Glucose to function efficiently and at their maximum potential, so the use of Fats should be considered very temporary.

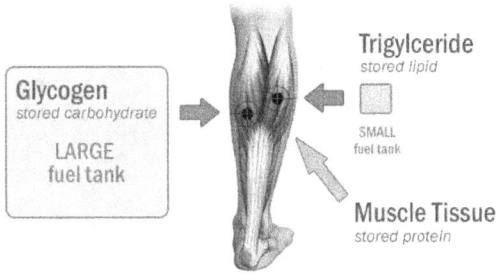

Body stores of Carbohydrates are relatively small but nevertheless serve as our most important LIFE Energy reserve.

An adult man has about 300 to 350 grams of Carbohydrates stored in his Liver and Muscles in the form of Glycogen. Another 10 grams of Glucose is in circulation in his Blood. Combined, both this Glycogen and Glucose have the power to supply the Energy needed for approximately a half day of moderate activity. To meet the body's constant demand, Carbohydrate foods must be eaten regularly and at reasonably frequent intervals.

CARBOHYDRATE STORAGE IN AN AVERAGE ADULT MAN
(70 kg [154 lb])

	GLYCOGEN (g)	GLUCOSE (g)
Liver	72	
Muscles	245	
Extracellular fluids		10
Component totals	317	10
total storage	327	

The body's 'fuel tanks'

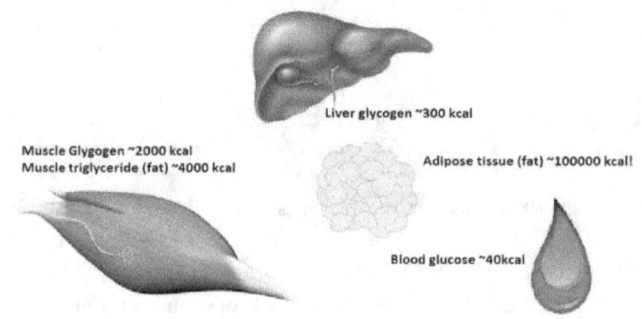

Liver glycogen ~300 kcal

Muscle Glygogen ~2000 kcal
Muscle triglyceride (fat) ~4000 kcal

Adipose tissue (fat) ~100000 kcal!

Blood glucose ~40kcal

Long-Term Sources of Energy

Long-term sources of Energy are dependent on the production of ATP from a variety of bio- fuels, with the primary element of Oxygen being required for utilization — which is the formation of Aerobic Energy. These primary bio-fuels include Muscle Glycogen, Blood Glucose, Plasma-free Fatty Acids, and Intramuscular Fats.

Protein only provides a small percentage of Energy needed to perform Muscle Contraction, so Carbs and Fats are our primary focus and sources that we need to ensure are adequately incorporated in our daily diet.

Glucose is broken-down and converted into Glycolysis (as described previously), and in this process the Pyruvic Acid is taken into the Mitochondria of our Cells, where it is then converted to a 2-Carbon fragment (Acetyl CoA) that enters the Krebs cycle. Fats are taken into the Mitochondria and they are also broken down into Acetyl CoA, which also enters the Krebs cycle. The energy originally contained in the Glucose and Fats is extracted from the Acetyl CoA and is used to generate ATP in the Electron Transport Chain that occurs in a process called *Oxidative Phosphorylation*, which requires Oxygen.

$$^* \textit{Carbohydrate and Fat} + O_2 \rightarrow ATP$$

ATP production performed through Aerobic mechanisms is slower than production from immediate and short-term sources of Energy, and when performing or completing submaximal work it may take 2 or 3 min before the ATP needs of the cell are completely fulfilled through the Aerobic process. The main reason for this longer extension of time is due to the time that it takes our Heart to increase the delivery of Oxygen-enriched Blood to our Muscles at the rate needed to meet the ATP demands of the Muscle to function/perform.

Aerobic production of ATP is the primary means of supplying LIFE Energy to our Muscles in maximal work lasting more than 2 min as well as in all submaximal work.

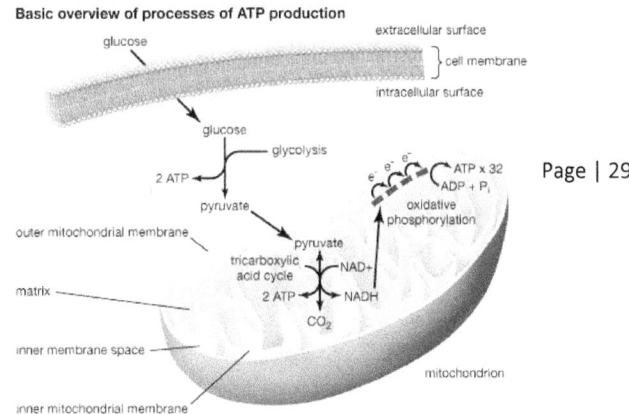

Basic overview of processes of ATP production

Taking place inside of our Cells, the Glucose is burned or metabolized to produce Heat and Adenosine Triphosphate (ATP), which is a Molecule that stores and releases Energy as required by the Cells to function. This transformation of Glucose into Energy occurs in one of two ways = With Oxygen or Without Oxygen.

Glucose is converted into Energy with the agency of Oxygen inside the Mitochondria, which are tiny bodies in the jellylike substance inside every Cell. This conversion yields LIFE Energy (ATP, Heat), the results of this Energy conversion manifests as Water and our waste product - Carbon Dioxide.

Since Red blood cells do not have Mitochondria, they convert Glucose into Energy without Oxygen which is Anaerobic. This process also yields LIFE Energy (ATP, Heat) in addition to Lactic Acid.

Within the fabric of our Muscle Cells is where Glucose is also converted to Energy. Muscle Cells have a Mitochondria, and because of which they can process and convert Glucose with Oxygen.

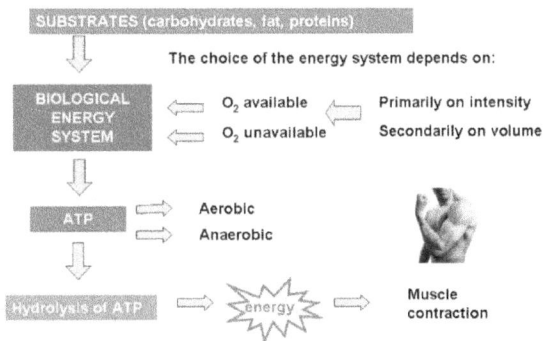

However, if or when the level of Oxygen in the Muscle Cell becomes deficient, the Muscle Cells can still temporarily convert (Anaerobic) Glucose into Energy without Oxygen.

This usually or most likely occurs during the performances of exercises so strenuously that you (and your muscles) are, literally, out of breath.

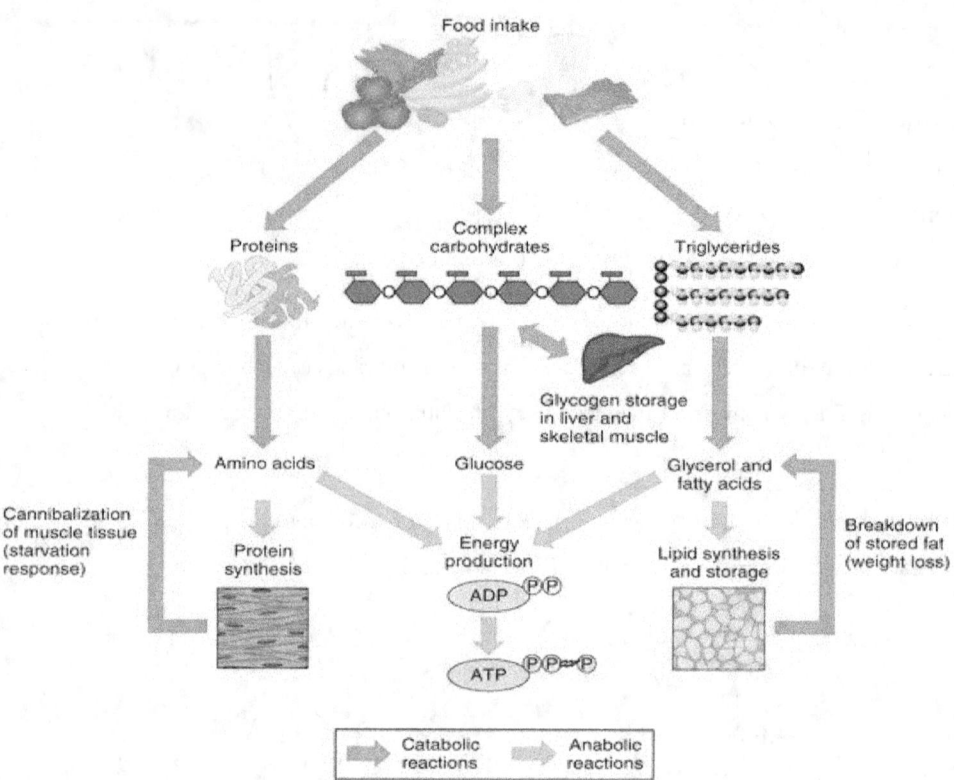

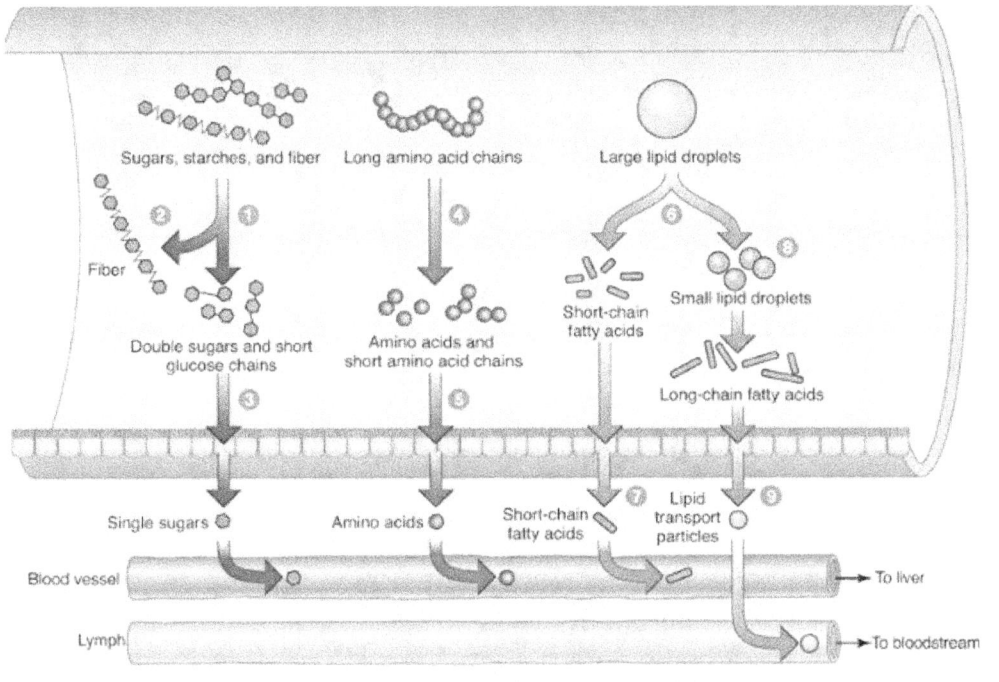

1. Pancreatic amylase digests starch to double sugars and short glucose chains.

2. Fiber, which cannot be digested by human enzymes, passes to the large intestine.

3. Enzymes in the microvilli digest double sugars into single sugars, which are absorbed into the blood.

4. Pancreatic proteases, along with proteases in the microvilli, digest long amino acid chains into amino acids and short amino acid chains.

5. Amino acids and short amino acid chains are absorbed into the mucosal cells, where they are digested into single amino acids, which pass into the blood.

6. Bile helps divide large fat globules. Pancreatic lipases digest fat molecules into fatty acids.

7. Short-chain fatty acids are absorbed into the mucosal cells and then pass directly into the blood.

8. Long-chain fatty acids and other lipids combine with bile to form small droplets that aid the absorption of fatty acids and other fat-soluble substances into the mucosal cell.

9. Absorbed lipids are incorporated into transport particles that pass into the lymph. They enter the blood without first passing through the liver.

Chapter 4: Special Functions

* * * * *

The elements of Carbohydrates have other specialized roles in our overall body Metabolism that extends well beyond its Nutritive properties which include the following:

Glycogen–Carbohydrate Storage. Liver and Muscle Glycogen are in a constant state of interchanging with our body's overall Energy system. These Energy reserves have several functions that include: protecting our Cells (particularly Brain Cells), from a depressed metabolic function and injury as well as offer support in urgent Muscle responses.

Protein-Sparing Action. Carbohydrates help regulate the metabolism of Protein. An adequate supply of Carbohydrate is required to satisfy our bodies constant Energy demands prevents the redirection of protein for Energy. This protein-sparing action of Carbs allows Protein to be utilized for and in its natural function of Tissue building and repair.

Antiketogenic Effect. Carbohydrates influence Fat metabolism. The supply of Carbohydrates determines how much Fat needs to be converted to meet our Energy needs, therefore controls the formation of Ketones. Ketones are small elements of Fat metabolism that normally are produced in very small amounts.

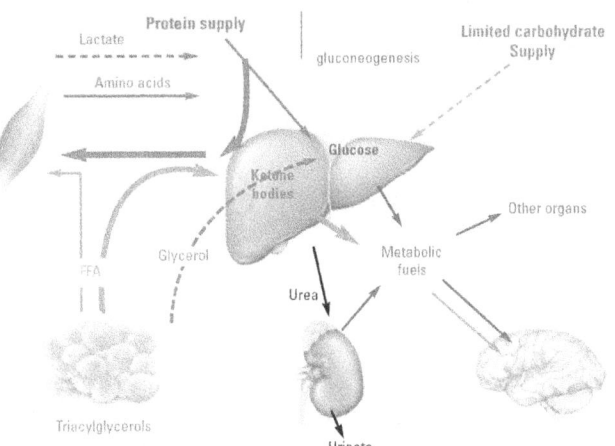

However, when our Carbohydrate supply is inadequate/deficient to meet our Cells Energy needs, which usually manifests from starvation or uncontrolled diabetes or very low-Carb diet.

Fat is oxidized at extreme rates and having sufficient amounts of dietary Carbohydrates prevent any damaging excess or build-up of Ketones.

Heart Action.

Heart action is a life-sustaining Muscle activity. Fatty Acids are the preferred Fuel/Energy for our Heart, where the Glycogen is stored in our Cardiac Muscle and additionally functions as an important emergency source of Contractile Energy.

A High intake of naturally occurring dietary Fiber is a major factor that's associated with creating a lower risk for Heart dis-ease.

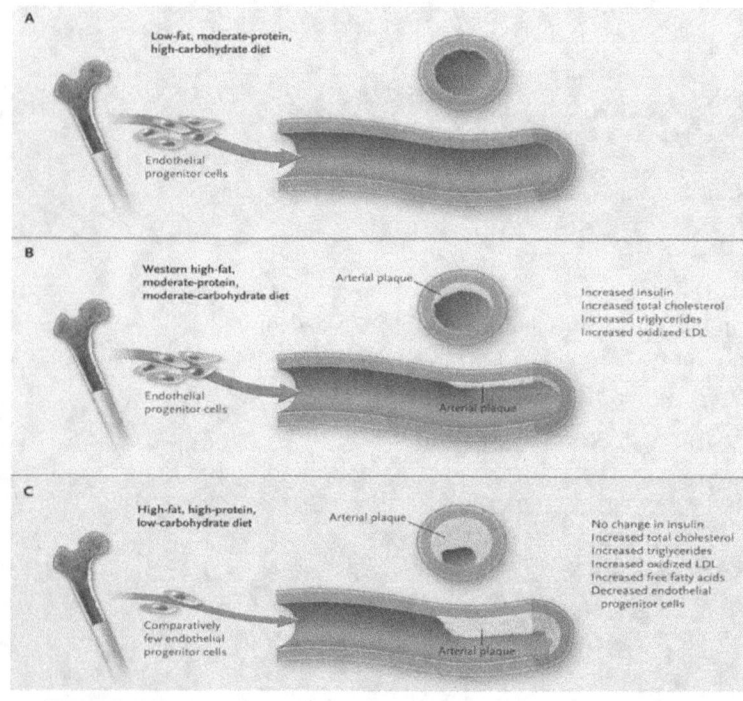

A higher intake of these dietary Fiber and Whole Grains are also important in the control and prevention of High Blood Pressure, high insulin levels, excess weight, high levels of Triglycerides, and low levels of HDL [good type] Cholesterol.

In the most recent research, the following results were concluded: several studies link dietary sugar with adverse changes in lipoproteins. Several studies have shown the existence of an inverse association between dietary sucrose and High-Density Lipoprotein (HDL) Cholesterol.

Data from the Coronary Artery Risk Development In young Adults (CARDIA) study shows a consistent inverse association between increased dietary Sucrose intake and HDL Cholesterol concentrations, in analyses in blacks and whites, in both men and women, and after adjustment for other co-varieies.

A diet high in Sucrose (over 20% of Energy) is associated with an elevation of Plasma Triglyceride concentrations. This increase is attributed to both an increased Hepatic secretion and impaired clearance of very-Low-Density Lipoprotein.

The Triglyceride response to dietary Sugar will usually vary and be altered according to the amount of Sugar and the presence of other Nutrients.

Central Nervous System. The Brain and Central Nervous System (CNS) depend on Carbohydrates for Energy but they have very low Carbohydrate reserves capacity—enough to last only 10 to 15 minutes. This makes these systems especially dependent on a minute-to-minute supply of Glucose from our Blood and increases the important role and function of Carbs as our primary source of LIFE Energy.

Glucose increases the synthesis of Acetylcholine, which is a Neurotransmitter that acts on areas of our Brain that's responsible for our Memory and Cognitive functions. This means that a Sharp, Crisp, Fast acting and operating Mind is built on Glucose.

Our Brain is our Control Center and where all body functions start. Our Brains is where we have the ability to overcome and control our Emotions and rise above them with Critical Thinking, which makes a diet that has the proper amount of Glucose included produces the Maximum Brain Power!

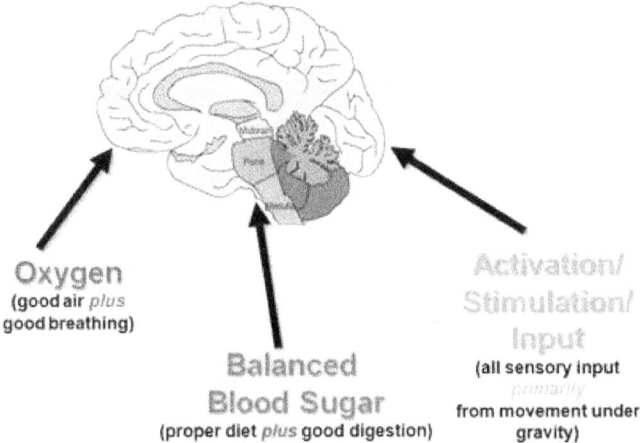

Oxygen
(good air *plus* good breathing)

Balanced
Blood Sugar
(proper diet *plus* good digestion)

Activation/
Stimulation/
Input
(all sensory input *primarily* from movement under gravity)

Chapter 5: Carbohydrates and Oral Health

* * * * *

Our Nutrient intake and Oral health have a synergistic relationship that works in both directions.

Malnutrition and other Nutrition-related diseases lead to deterioration and decay of our Teeth and supporting Tissues of the Mouth and Gums to the point that eating becomes difficult and the level of Nutrient intake is decreased further.

Conversely, the different infectious diseases that present in the Mouth, like untreated as well as a case

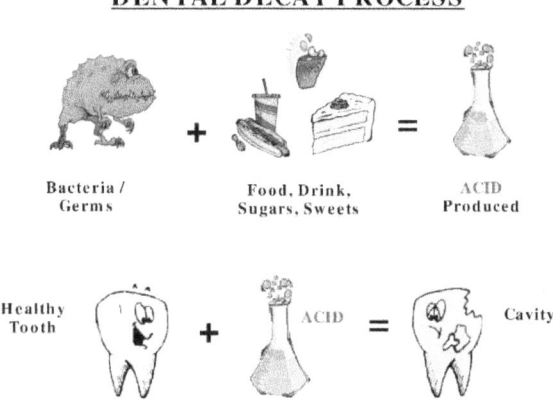

DENTAL DECAY PROCESS

Bacteria / Germs + Food, Drink, Sugars, Sweets = ACID Produced

Healthy Tooth + ACID = Cavity

of progressive periodontal disease, result in systemic infections and hampers the bodies ability of Glucose control in relation to diabetes. Also there is an increase in inflammatory responses and cardiovascular risk.

Dental Caries are one of the most frequently occurring as well as preventable infectious diseases that manifest in our oral cavity and is major factor of Tooth loss.

Oral hygiene, diet, and specific Nutrients have been shown to be related to cause of Dental Caries.

Over- exposure to Fluoride that we consume in the form of fluoridated water or fluoride treatments results in an increase in the erosion of Tooth Enamel that is less resistant to bacterial action and decay. Those that reside in areas where their water is Fluoridated have an 18% higher rate of Dental Caries than those who have little to no exposure to Fluoridation.

The amounts and types of dietary Carbohydrates and in conjunction with the conditions under which they are eaten have a serious impact on the formation of Dental Caries. Bacteria in the Dental Plaque ferment both naturally occurring and added (manufactured/processed) Sugars and Short-Chain Starch Molecules to form Acid. This action causes the effect on a drop in our pH level and creates an Acidic environment in self which favors the action of the *55Streptococci* strain of Bacteria that initial cause of Dental Caries.

MICROBIOLOGY OF DENTAL CARIES

Caries:

Localized destruction of the tissues of the tooth by bacterial fermentation of dietary carbohydrates

A multifactorial, plaque-related chronic infection of the enamel, cementum or dentine

Children and adolescents who consume higher amounts of added (processed/manufactured) Sugar have a documented increase of Dental Caries.

Naturally occurring Sugars also can also lead to tooth decay, but we also have an abundance of Plants that contribute to Tooth health like Citrus Fruits that are composed of a high proportion of Water, that in addition to Citric Acid, helps to stimulate our Salivary secretion which aids in rinsing our Teeth and help remove Sugars (natural and un-natural) from the surface of the Tooth's Enamel.

The length of exposure to a sweet solution also drastically affects its Cariogenic potential. Continuously sipping on Sugar-sweetened beverages throughout the day dramatically increases the risk of Tooth Caries and Decay.

Prevention of these Dental Caries should be yet another reason for us to wisely recognize and choose Whole-Grain Breads and Cereals over the consumption of highly processed grains and grain foods with added (processed/manufactured) Sugar.

Unprocessed Starch manifests as a large Molecule that cannot pass through the Dental Plaque to attack the Enamel, however, the shorter-chain Oligosaccharides are more easily converted by our Salivary Amylase to create Maltose, which is a primary choice substrate (food) for Plaque Bacteria.

Grain-sugar mixtures, such as ready-to-eat breakfast cereals or cakes, are especially Cariogenic.

Foods High in Sugar

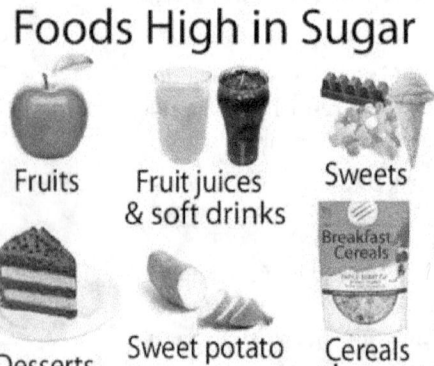

Fruits

Fruit juices & soft drinks

Sweets

Desserts

Sweet potato

Cereals ready-to-eat

Chronic disease increases an individual's vulnerability to Dental Caries and the resultant Tooth loss. Age-related loss of calcium from the bones (or the drastic bone loss occurring in osteoporosis) affects the Alveolar Bone also resulting in Tooth loss.

A Reduction of the production of Salivary secretion (dry mouth) is closely associated with Diabetes and with particular medications accelerates both Tooth decay and damage to our Oral Tissues.

Dental caries can also result from poor dental hygiene and continuous snacking and drinking of items high in added sugar or other refined carbohydrates.

(From Mahan LK, Escott-Stump S: *Krause's food and nutrition therapy,* ed 12, St Louis, Mo., 2008, Saunders.)

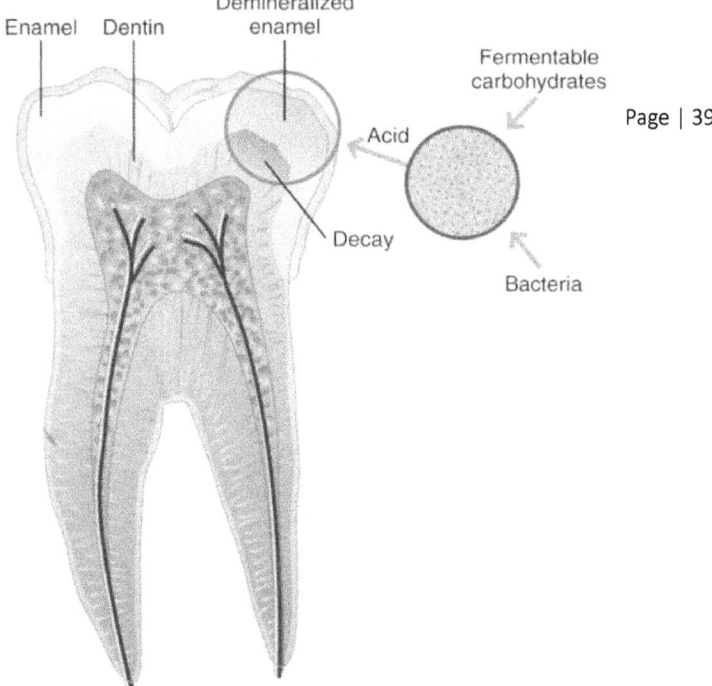

FIGURE 3-2   Dental caries can result from poor dental hygiene and continuous snacking and drinking of items high in added sugar or other refined carbohydrates. (From Mahan LK, Escott-Stump S: *Krause's food and nutrition therapy,* ed 12, St Louis, Mo., 2008, Saunders.)

Chapter 6: Weight Management

* * * * *

As the popularity of low-carb diets have increased, it has come at the cost of ALL Carbohydrates in general gaining a negative reputation of being unhealthy and fattening. The reality is that it's consumption of food like products that are made from Refined and processed Carbs that are DEVOID LIFE Energy of the SUN.

In general, naturally occurring Carbs present no more fattening properties than any other Nutrient and there is no evidence that even suggests or supports that the proportion of our total Carb intake in our diet has any effect on Energy intake or Body weight.

Weight gain is a product of Cause and Effect. The gain in weight is the Effect that is experienced by the direct Cause of an excessive consumption of K Calories - with no regards to whether these excessive Kcals derive from Carbohydrates, Fats, or Proteins.

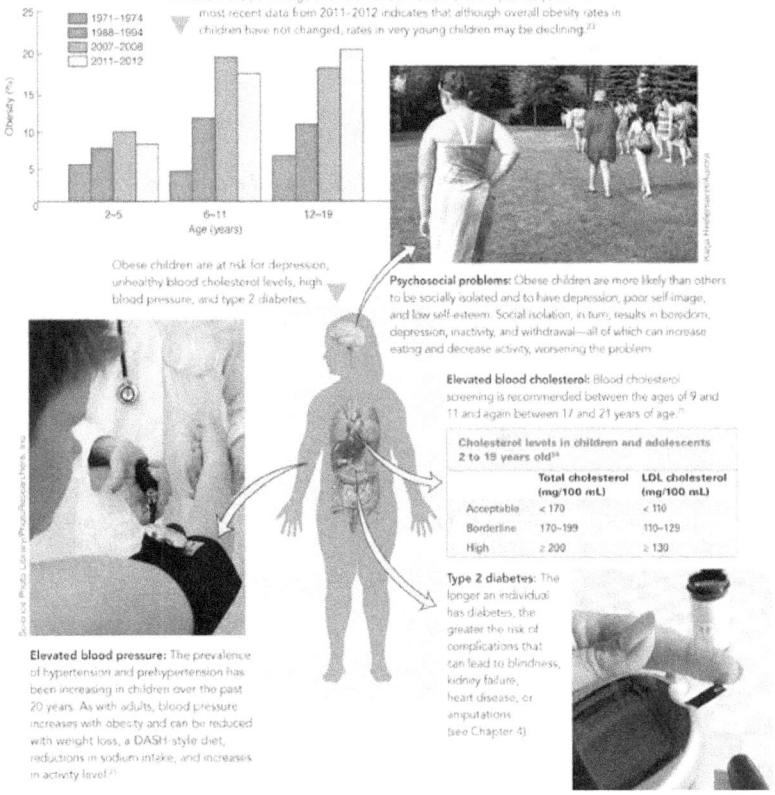

In perspective, Carbohydrates provide only 4 KCalories per gram which are less than half of the 9 KCalories per gram provided by Fat.

Carbohydrates and weight loss

After finishing a meal, the type of Carbohydrates that we consumed in that meal are the direct

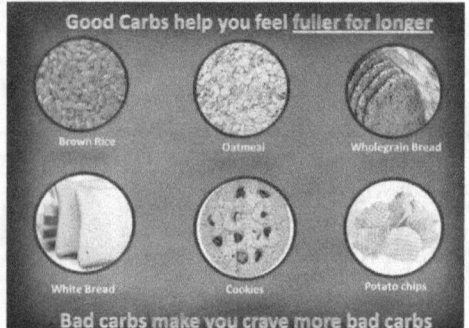

Cause which determines the Effect of how hungry you feel and how soon we feel hungry again after we eat. Both of these are determining factors to whether we LOSE or GAIN weight.

A Diet that's high in UNREFINED (naturally occurring) Carbs is also high in Unrefined dietary Fiber, which creates to the direct Cause of a sense of fullness by adding bulk and slowing digestion, both of which are responsible for the Effect of allowing us to feel satisfied and full with less food.

This is the natural formula to help promote Healthy weight-loss, as well as Naturally maintaining our proper weight.

However, it most be noted that diets high in Fiber may be problematic for children, who have a small stomach capacity, because they may become satiated before meeting all their Nutritional requirements.

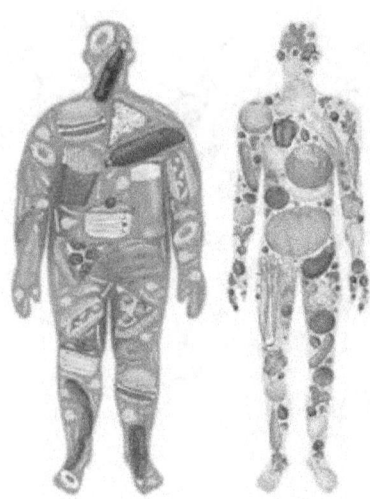

Beverages and Energy Intake

A diet that high in the Unnatural/processed sugar-sweetened beverages will have an immediate and detrimental increase their Caloric intake, but these beverages do not induce satiety or fullness to the same extent as solid foods.

Also, several studies show and support the fact that increases in the consumption of these types of sugar-sweetened soft drinks are closely associated with weight GAIN. Not to mention the wide-ranging other health issues that is directly associated with these sugar-sweetened beverages.

We are comprised of approximately 75% Water, and even though these sugar-sweetened drinks are water-based LIQUIDS – THEY ARE NOT WATER.

WE ARE WHAT WE DRINK !!!!

Foods high in REFINED/Un-Natural Carbohydrates cause an immediate rise in Blood Glucose and this action causes the reaction of the stimulation and release of Insulin.

Learning how to balance your intake of carbs can keep your body fueled while you manage to lose weight.

Good Carbs | Bad Carbs
Vegetables
Fruits
Whole Grains
Seeds
Nuts
Beans

In our bodies, Insulin promotes Fat storage. Which means that a diet high in REFINED/Un-Natural Carbs will be the catalyst that Causes more-than-normal Insulin release, which will manifest in the detrimental Effect of shifting our Metabolism towards Fat storage (Potential Energy) instead out natural action of Fat burning (Kinetic Energy).

In contrast, a low-Carbohydrate (consisting of foods low in naturally occurring Carbs) diet causes a condition of having deficient Insulin release and the opposite reaction occurs, which does not promote Fat storage.

Low-Carb diets mainly leads to Weight Loss because these diets severely limit the food choices to such an extent that the monotony of the diet may just cause the dieter to eat less.

It's Very Important to be mindful that the weight loss that is achieved with these diets is therefore only caused by the consuming fewer calories and not necessarily from a healthy perspective.

Especially since we know that Carbohydrates are our 1st and primary source of LIFE Energy.

Imbalances in Carbohydrate Intake

Simple CHO
i)   glucose sugars naturally found in fruits and honey, cane sugar/ table sugar & milk sugar , added sugar in foods such as soft drinks and cakes

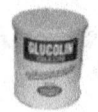  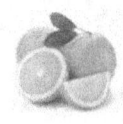 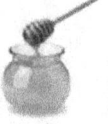 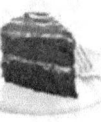 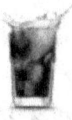

Complex CHO
i)   Starches(eg: rice, oats, breads, potatoes, yam corn, peas, grains, cereal)

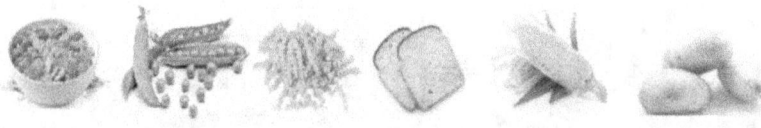

ii)   Fibers (mainly found in brown rice, wholegrain products, barley, fruits, most vegetables, oats)

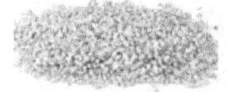 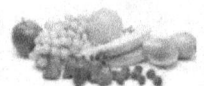 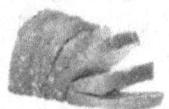 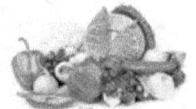

High-Carbohydrate Diets

The recommendations for our Carbohydrate intake is approximately 45% to 65% of our total Energy. A high-Carb diet is when an someone has increased their Carbs intake to 75% with purpose of trying simultaneously lower their intakes of Fat and KCals or attempting to normalize Blood Lipoproteins with this higher intake of Carbs.

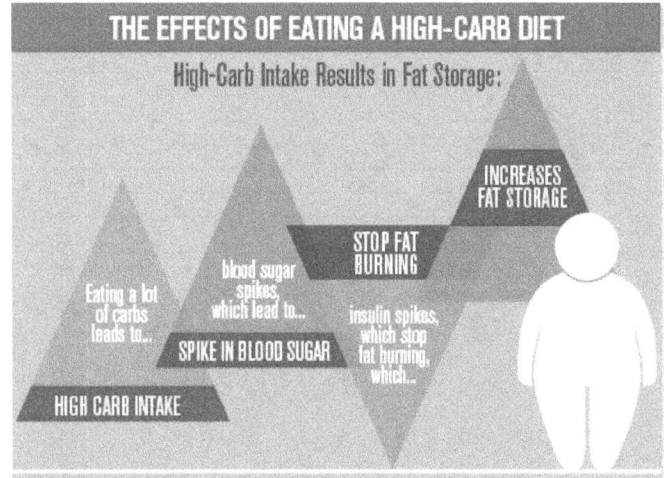

When our Carb intake exceeds 65% of our total KCalories, it means that our Fat intake becomes disproportionately low, which causes the reaction of jeopardizing our necessary supply of Essential Fatty Acids and Vitamins and Minerals that are found in higher-Fat foods that we also may consume.

An increase like this in dietary Carbs can trigger a rise in Plasma Triglycerides and **Low-Density Lipoprotein (LDL) Cholesterol**, and a drop in **High-Density Lipoprotein (HDL) Cholesterol**, which dangerously increases chances of Cardiovascular risk.

Excessive Carb intake, with a high dis-proportion of Simple Carbohydrates or added Sugars, brings about rapid elevations in Blood Glucose, which places an unhealthy heavy demand on the Pancreas for Insulin production and release.

Whole-Grain foods, Legumes, or Fruits and Veggies that are naturally high in Fiber and other Complex Carbohydrates are better choices when attempting to increase intake because they represent the best sources of naturally occurring Carbs/Fiber.

The following graph shows the approximate Time it takes our Bodies to deplete our Stores of Energy in the form of Nutrients.

Our Carbohydrates are Depleted within 13 Hours!

Other than Amino Acids, EVERY other Nutrient takes DAYS for us to Deplete!!!

So, a diet that provides the necessary amount of Carbohydrates, keeps us at Maximum Energy Levels and Surplus. Carbs are our Main and Preferred Source of LIFE ENERGY!!!

EXTENT OF BODY RESERVES OF NUTRIENTS

NUTRIENT	TIME REQUIRED TO DEPLETE RESERVES IN WELL-NOURISHED INDIVIDUALS
Amino acids	Several hours
Carbohydrate	13 hours
Sodium	2-3 days
Water	4 days
Zinc	5 days
Fat	20-40 days
Thiamin	30-60 days
Vitamin C	60-120 days
Niacin	60-180 days
Riboflavin	60-180 days
Vitamin A	90-365 days
Iron	125 days (women), 750 days (men)
Iodine	1000 days
Calcium	2500 days

From Guthrie HA: *Introductory nutrition*, ed 7, St Louis, Mo., 1989, Mosby.

Low-Carbohydrate Diets

Diets very low in Carbohydrates have been popularized as efficient ways to lose weight. Such diets may restrict Carbohydrate intake to 130 grams or less, often equaling 10% or less of total KCalories, dangerously lower than the RDI. These regimens bring about weight loss over the short term *ONLY IF* the Energy intake is also reduced ALONG WITH have a favorable effect of these specific Metabolic parameters including Blood LDL Cholesterol, HDL Cholesterol, and Triglycerides.

There are several questions that remain as to their appropriateness when followed for weeks or months. It is important that all dietary patterns include the minimum daily servings of fruits, vegetables, and whole grains and any dietary plan that alters the respective percentage should be thoroughly researched as to its validity and safety.

These Plant-based Carbohydrate foods also supply health-promoting naturally occurring Nutrients and Fiber and assist in our ability of controlling our Blood Pressure.

Low-Carb diets that replace these naturally occurring Carbohydrate foods with food-like items that are high in Saturated Fat are the underlying cause of Cardiovascular dis-ease and risk. Low-Carb diets that replace these Carbohydrates with Protein exceeding AMDR levels increase the burden on the Kidneys and most people that follow a low-Carb diet have Kidney problems.

A Healthier approach to reducing ones Carbohydrate intake is by eliminating food-like items that are high in sugar, such as sugar-sweetened beverages and baked items, and reserving your Carb intake for Fruits, Vegetables and Whole Grains.

A low-carbohydrate diet changes the Energy currency that's available to our Cells from Glucose to Fatty-Acids, this is health-dangerous because the Cells of our Central Nervous System (CNS) is always dependent on Glucose and a steady supply of it.

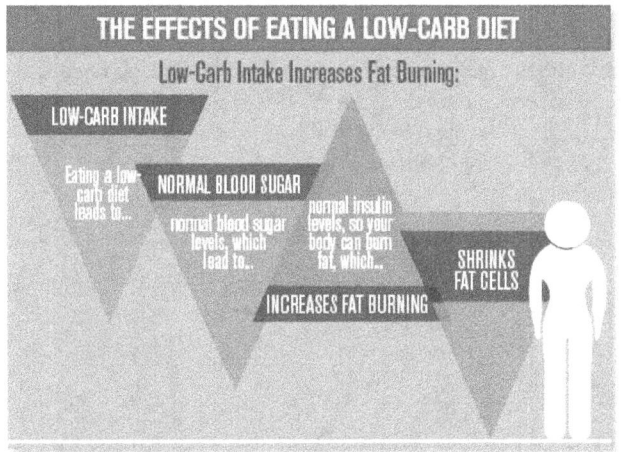

This change in body Metabolism from the results of a low-Carb diet has proven useful in the treatment of several chronic conditions and especially effective in lowering Blood Glucose levels in some people with Diabetes - although severe Carbohydrate restriction (below 45% of total KCalories) is generally not recommended and warned against. Usually those that suffer from Diabetes is from the result of eating refined, manufactured and processed Carbs and after years of eating this way it makes our Bodies reject naturally occurring Carbohydrates and can only Metabolize a little at a time.

The accelerated breakdown of Fat for Energy, which produces Ketones, CAUSES an anticonvulsant EFFECT. The resulting Ketosis from consuming a low-Carb diet can also assist in the management of nonalcoholic fatty liver disease, certain cancers, and neurodegenerative conditions, such as Alzheimer's and Parkinson's diseases.

*** *Note that the Ketosis as discussed here is significantly different from Ketoacidosis, which is a potentially fatal condition Manifesting from the condition of uncontrolled diabetes.* ***

However, even moderate a mild state of Ketosis increases Water loss, necessitating attention to Water intake, taking care to maintain proper Hydration. When Glucose is in short supply, Amino Acids are then broken down to provide the necessary Carbon Skeletons for Glucose Synthesis, which produces Amino groups that must be disposed of via the Urine.

The Nutritional elements Calcium and Potassium are also lost in this process so adequate intakes of both becomes critical.

The apparent safety and effectiveness of low-carbohydrate diets with appropriate medical supervision supports the need for more than one dietary approach to weight control, adapted to individual preferences and metabolic needs.

Regardless, establishing a KCalorie deficit between Energy intake and Energy expenditure using a combination of foods that support our Nutritional well-being is the ONLY cornerstone of long-term weight management and health.

Understanding Carbohydrates: Life Energy, Fiber, Sugar & Starch!

Weight-loss diets based on the glycemic index typically recommend limiting foods that are higher on the Glycemic Index which normally and Foods with this high ranking include Potatoes and Corn, and manufactured and processed food-like items such as snack foods and desserts that contain refined flours and sugars. Many healthy foods, such as Whole Grains, Legumes, Vegetables, Fruits and Whole Milk and Whole Milk Dairy products, are naturally lower on the Glycemic Index.

GLYCEMIC INDEX OF COMMON CARBOHYDRATE FOODS*

FOOD	GLYCEMIC INDEX
Glucose test dose (50 g)	100
Baked potato (without skin)	98
Corn flakes	80
Jelly beans	80
Bread, white	77
Cupcake, frosted	73
Spaghetti	65
Banana	62
Bread, whole wheat	59
Orange juice	54
Green peas	51
Apple	39
White rice, long grain	38
All-bran cereal	38
Milk, nonfat	37
Kidney beans, canned	36
Fructose	15

*The test dose of 50 g glucose is assigned the value of 100 and serves as the standard to evaluate other foods.

Data from Atkinson FS, Foster-Powell K, Brand-Miller JC: International Tables of Glycemic Index and Glycemic Load Values. *Diab Care* 31(12):2281, 2008. (Supplementary Table A1; available online.)

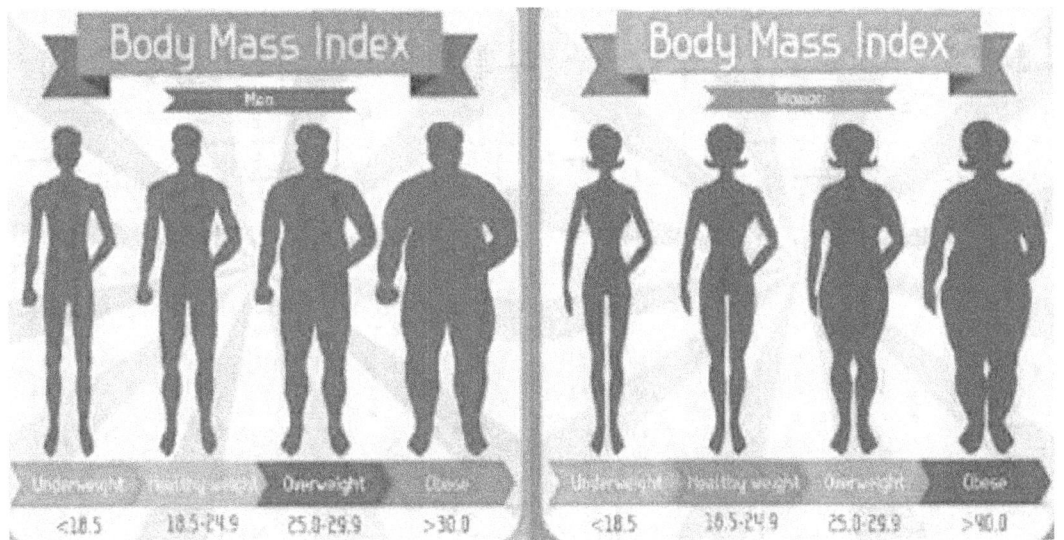

Chapter 7: Understanding Carbs

*****

A Carbohydrate is a Nutrient that's composed of Carbon, Hydrogen, and Oxygen and is the Essential source of Energy in and for the body.

Carbs can be divided into three categories: Monosaccharides, Disaccharides, and Polysaccharides. Examples of Monosaccharides are Glucose and Fructose.

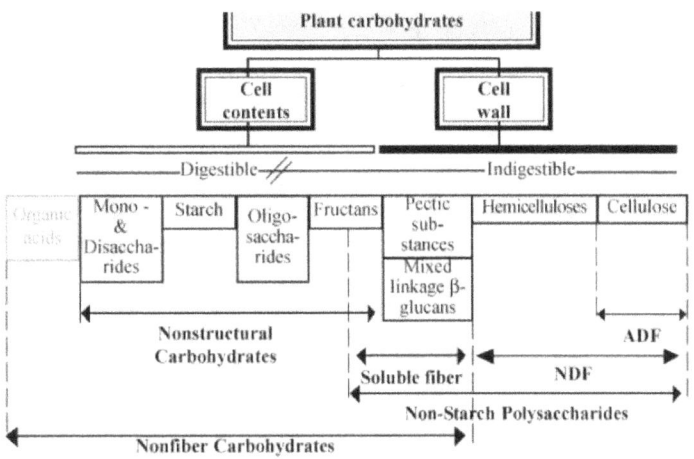

Carbohydrates that form from the combining of 2 Monosccharides are called Disaccharides. Lactose and Sucrose are two of the Disaccharides. Both the Monosaccharides and Disaccharides are sometimes called Simple Sugars. Simple Sugars contribute significantly to the Caloric content of food-like items such as fruit juices, soft drinks, and candy.

The most important Simple Sugar in the Human Body is manifested in the form of Glucose.

The Molecular formula for Glucose is $C_6H_{12}O_6$. Polysaccharides are Complex Carbs that are formed by combining three or more Sugar Molecules. Starches and Fiber are Polysaccharides found in plants. Whole-grain and the products made from them breads are high in Complex Carbs.

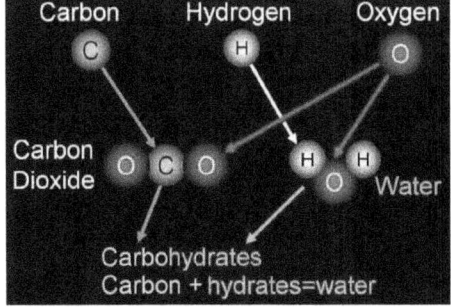

When Carbohydrates are stored in the body, Glucose Molecules begin to join together to form large Molecules called Glycogen. Glycogen is stored in the liver and skeletal muscle.

Grains, Vegetables, and Fruits are excellent sources of **Carbohydrate**. It is recommended that 45% to 65% of a person's daily calories come from Carbs. The majority of our dietary Carb KCalories should derive from Complex Carbohydrates while food-like items with added sugar should be avoided.

The reason for eating Complex rather than Simple Carbs is the higher Nutrient density of Complex Carbs. Nutrient Density refers to the amount of Essential Nutrients that's Bio-available in a specific food compared with the KCalories it contains. As an example, a candy bar (containing Simple Sugars) has a Low Nutrient Density, whereas a slice of whole-grain bread (containing Complex Carbs) has a Hgh Nutrient Density.

One of the simultaneous benefits of consuming foods that are high in naturally occurring in Complex Carbs is that they also typically contain naturally occurring dietary Fiber, which is a non-Starch Polysaccharide that is found in Plants and cannot be digested by our Digestive system. Although this Fiber cannot be digested, it helps prevent hemorrhoids, constipation, and cancers of the Digestive system by helping to move food quickly and easily through our Digestive System which prevents rot and fermentation. In addition, consuming Water-Soluble Fiber has been shown to lower Cholesterol levels.

Unfortunately, the typical American diet is low in naturally occurring Fiber, with the average intake being approximately 15 grams a day. The AI for our dietary Fiber intake for men and women aged 50 and younger is 38 and 25 grams a day respectively. For older men and women with lower calorie consumption, the daily recommended levels are 30 g and 21 g, respectively.

Dietary Guidelines for Americans, 2010 recommends that adults consume approximately 14 grams of naturally occurring Fiber for every 1,000 KCals consumed.

Excellent sources of naturally occurring dietary Fiber are Whole Grains, Vegetables, Legumes, and Fruits.

Carbohydrates (carbs) provide **Glucose!**
Glucose from carbs gives our body **ENERGY!**

Glucose provides:

- The **only** source of energy for the brain.

- The primary source of energy for the heart and skeletal muscles.

- When the athlete's body runs out of glucose, their muscles fatigue and performance declines QUICKLY.

Carbohydrates are a vital source of LIFE Energy in and for the Human Body. During high-intensity exercise, Carbohydrates are the primary fuel source for ATP production. When Carbs are metabolized in the human body, it yields approximately 4 KCals of Energy per gram. This means that a person who eats 10 grams of Carbs gain approximately 40 KCals of LIFE Energy to use or store.

Basic Fuels: Sugars and Starch

There are 2 forms of digestible **Carbohydrates** that occur naturally in Plant Foods: (1) Sugars and (2) Starch. All Energy on our planet Earth comes ultimately from the Sun and its action on the Plants. The Sun not only supplies the Life Energy for us here on Earth, it is the LIFE Energy (second to POWER of The CREATOR) for ALL in the Universe, from the single Atom to Planets.

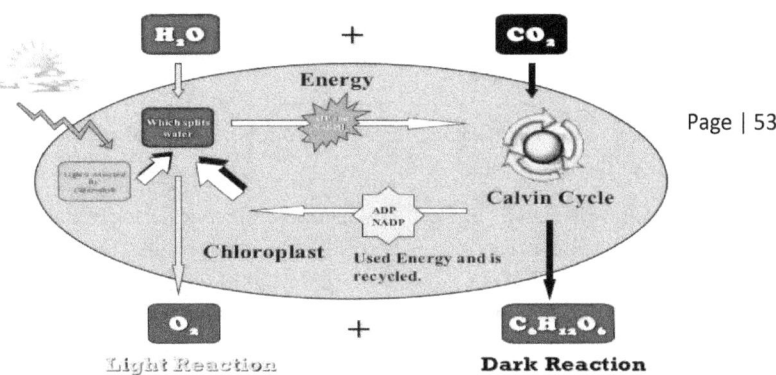

Using their internal process of Photosynthesis, the Plants/Vegetation transforms the Sun's LIFE Energy into the stored fuel known as Carbohydrates.

Nothing leaves the Atmosphere of our Planet, which means that everything is literally recycled, including our Breath. These Plants use our Carbon Dioxide (CO_2), in conjunction with the Energy from the Life Elements of Air, Water and Soil to manifest Chlorophyll (Plant Pigment) -the chemical catalyst to manufacture and manifest Sugars and Starch.

These Carbohydrates that the Plants manufacture, they also store for their own Energy needs now becomes the major source of LIFE Fuel for humans, whose primary food are Plants. Because our bodies can rapidly break down Starch and Sugars - Carbohydrates are often referred to as *Quick Energy Foods.* ***They are our primary source of energy***.

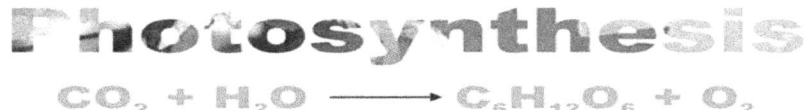

$$CO_2 + H_2O \longrightarrow C_6H_{12}O_6 + O_2$$

Description 1: The process in green plants and certain other organisms by which carbohydrates are synthesized from carbon dioxide and water using light as an energy source. Most forms of photosynthesis release oxygen as a byproduct. (The Free Dictionary)

$$6CO_2 + 12H_2O \longrightarrow C_6H_{12}O_6 + 6O_2 + 6H_2O$$

Description 2: The process by which some cells in green plants are able to trap light energy and use it to split the Hydrogen and Oxygen in water. The Oxygen is given off, and the Hydrogen is combined with Carbon and Oxygen from CO_2 to make simple sugars, which are used as a food source immediately, or combined to make starch, or used in the manufacture of other substances. The light energy used is not green – green light is not absorbed by chlorophyll. Chlorophyll and other pigments trap the light, and the cell uses enzymes to split water, and to synthesize the products of photosynthesis. The energy-providing food we eat comes, directly or indirectly, from photosynthesis.

Dietary Importance

Carbohydrates make up a major portion of the food of people all over the world. Fruits, vegetables, cereals, grains, and dairy foods supply Carbs and in some countries fruits, vegetables, and grains make up approximately 85% of the diet.

Rice has become one of the world's most important sources of Carbohydrates, used in the feeding of 3 billion people in the developing world.

In the typical American diet, about one half of total Kilocalories (KCalories or KCal) come from refined grains that make what's considered BAD Carbohydrates. The Carbohydrates in these food-related items are BAD because they are devoid of the Energy of the SUN. Unfortunately, these Toxic products are readily available, relatively low in cost, and easily stored.

Compared with food items that require refrigeration or have a short shelf life, many Carbohydrate foods can be held in dry storage for fairly long periods without spoiling. Modern processing and packaging methods have unnaturally extended the shelf life of these BAD Carb products almost indefinitely with the aide of preservatives that release TOXIC ENERGY that causes damage to every Organ that it interacts with. This TOXIC Energy is known as a FREE-RADICAL.

These Free-Radicals cause damage to the DNA at a Cellular level, manifesting in the condition called Cancer.

If we only ate according to our Digestive System function, we would eliminate 99% of ALL Dis-eases, sicknesses and causes of Pre-Mature DEATH!!!

We would then have the Perfect environment WITHIN Self to Build our Supreme Health!

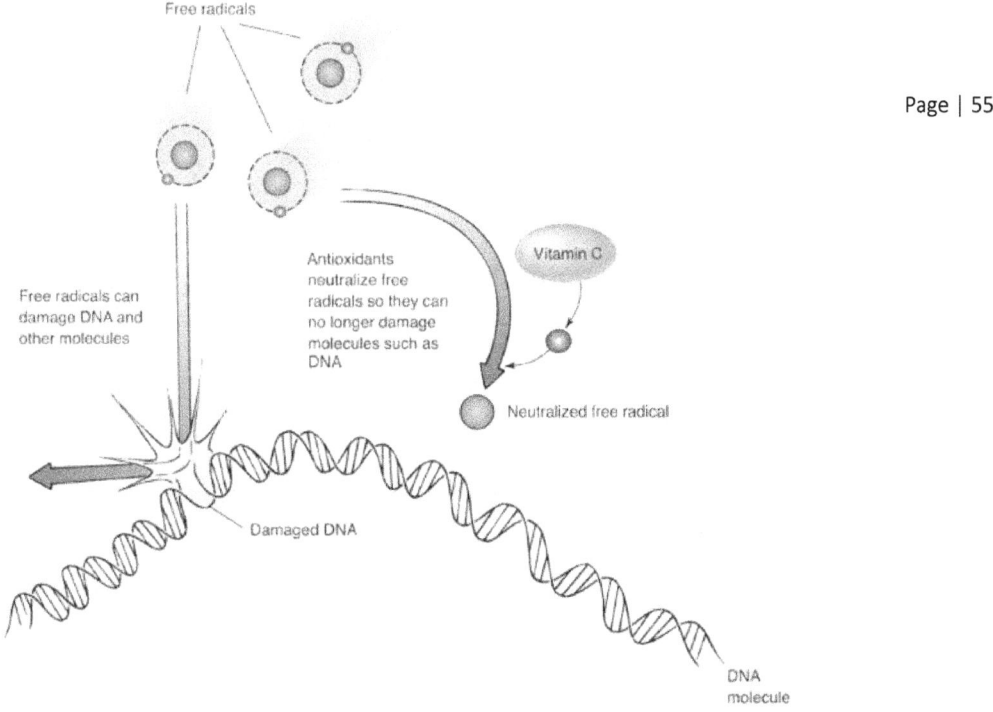

Chapter 8: Digestion of Carbs

* * * * *

Carbohydrate digestion begins in the Mouth, but most Starch digestion and the metabolizing of Disaccharides occur in our Small Intestines. The Carbs that cannot be digested then pass into the Colon. Some of this is broken down by Bacteria. The material that cannot be absorbed is excreted in our feces.

Digestion

The conversion of Starch and Sugars to Glucose starts in our Mouths where Salivary **Amylase** (Ptyalin) from our Parotid Gland acts on the Starch to begin transforming it into Dextrins and Maltose. There isn't a specific Enzyme in our Stomachs which acts on these Carbs, however, by the time the food mass is completely mixed with Gastric Acid, as much as 20% to 30% of the Starch has been broken down to Maltose. The Enzymes that complete the Chemical Digestion of these Carbohydrates come from two sources: our Pancreas and our Small Intestine.

• *Pancreatic secretions:* Pancreatic Amylase entering our Duodenum through our common Bile Duct completes the metabolizing of Starch to Maltose.

• *Intestinal secretions:* Cells within the brush border of our Small Intestine secretes three Disaccharides = **Sucrase**, **Lactase**, and **Maltase**, which act on their respective Disaccharides to release the Monosaccharides, Glucose, Galactose, and Fructose.

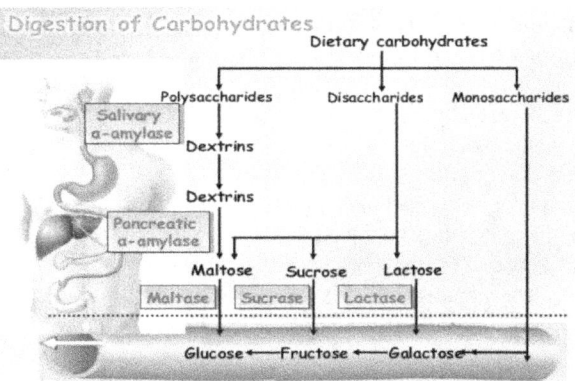

Understanding Carbohydrates: Life Energy, Fiber, Sugar & Starch!

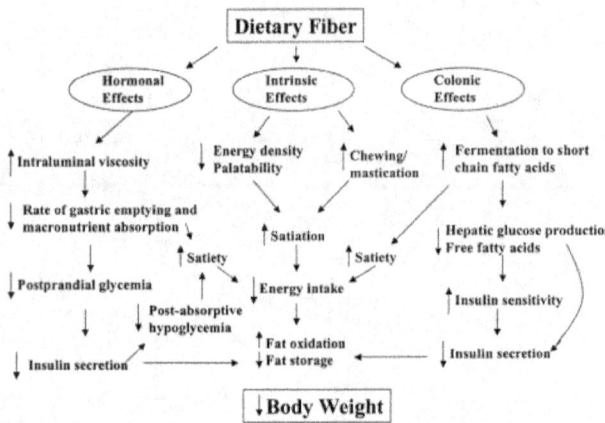

Absorption and Metabolism

Glucose is absorbed in our Bodies by an active pumping system that utilizes the element Sodium as a carrier.

Of the total Carbs that are absorbed, approximately 80% is now presented in the form of Glucose, leaving the remaining 20% manifested between the elements Galactose and Fructose.

By way of the Capillaries in our Villi, the by-products of this Carb digestion then enters our Blood circulation being routed to our Liver. Once at our Liver, the Fructose and Galactose are converted to Glucose.

The Glucose not needed for our immediate Energy needs is then converted to Glycogen or Adipose Tissue for storage which is Potential Energy.

Glucose can be used to provide Energy, which is stored as Liver Glycogen, or delivered via the general Blood circulation to other Body Tissues, causing Blood Glucose levels to rise.

Glycemic Response is a measure of the impact a food has on our Blood Glucose levels. How quickly and how high our Blood Glucose levels rise are affected by how long it takes a food to leave the Stomach and by how fast the food is digested as well as the Glucose absorbed.

Glycemic Response is the Rate, Magnitude, and Duration of the rise in Blood Glucose that occurs after food is consumed.

The Glycemic Index

A lower glycemic index suggests slower rates of digestion and absorption of the foods' carbohydrates and may also indicate greater extraction from the liver and periphery of the products of carbohydrate digestion. A lower glycemic response usually equates to a lower insulin demand but not always, and may improve long-term blood glucose control and blood lipids. The insulin index is also useful, as it provides a direct measure of the insulin response to a food.

Refined sugars and starches are the root cause of a greater Glycemic Response than unrefined Carbohydrates because the Sugars and Starches consumed alone leave the Stomach quickly and are rapidly digested and absorbed.

For example, when you drink a bottle of sugary soda, your Blood Glucose increases within minutes. Because Fiber takes longer to leave the Stomach and slows absorption in the Small Intestine, a Fiber-containing food such as oatmeal would take longer to leave your Stomach and therefore cause a lower Glycemic Response.

When Carbohydrates, Fats, and Proteins are consumed together, the emptying of our Stomachs is slowed, which causes a delay of both digestion and absorption of these Carbs, so our Blood Glucose rises more slowly than when these Carbs are consumed alone.

For instance, after a meal of chicken, brown rice, and green beans, which contains Carbs, Fats, Protein, and Fiber, the Blood Glucose wouldn't begin to increase for approximately 30 to 60 minutes after consumption.

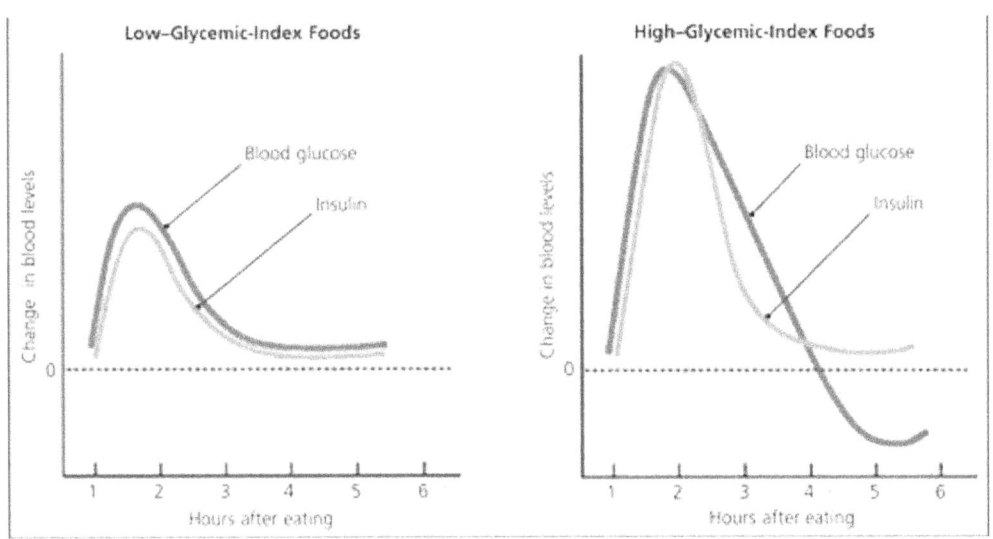

Glycemic response to 100g food

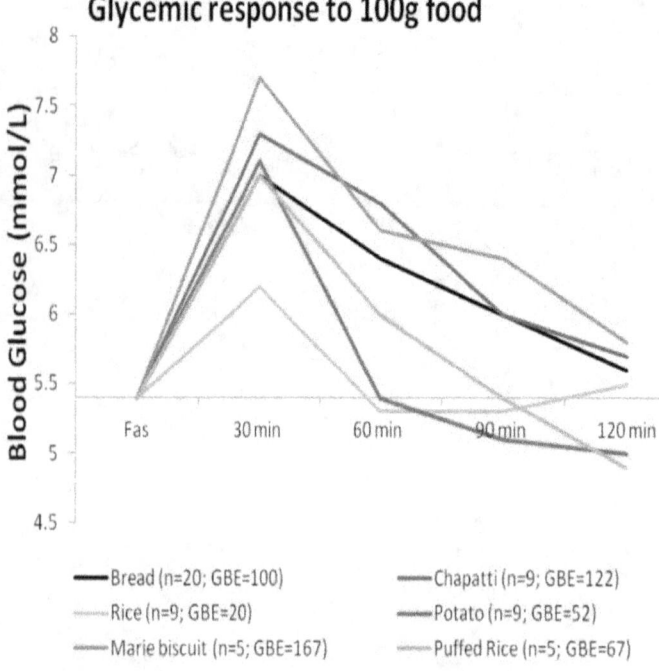

Bread (n=20; GBE=100)

Chapatti (n=9; GBE=122)

Rice (n=9; GBE=20)

Potato (n=9; GBE=52)

Marie biscuit (n=5; GBE=167)

Puffed Rice (n=5; GBE=67)

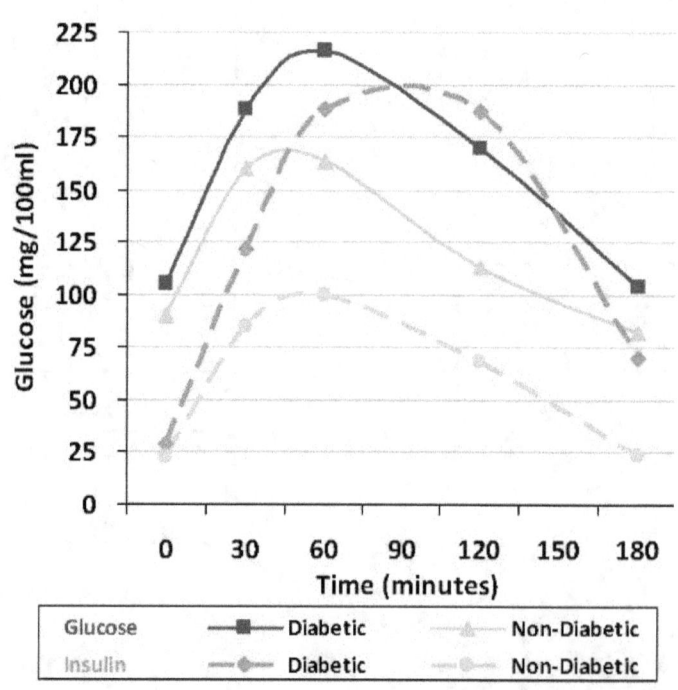

| Glucose | Diabetic | Non-Diabetic |
| Insulin | Diabetic | Non-Diabetic |

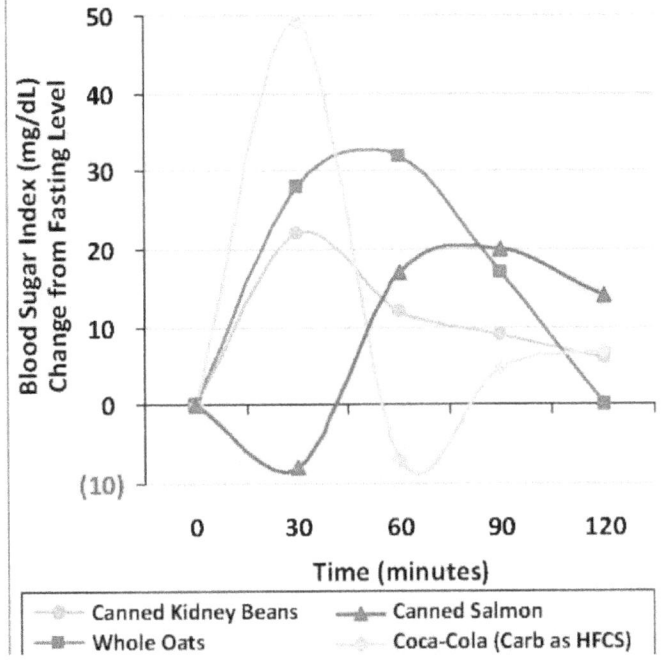

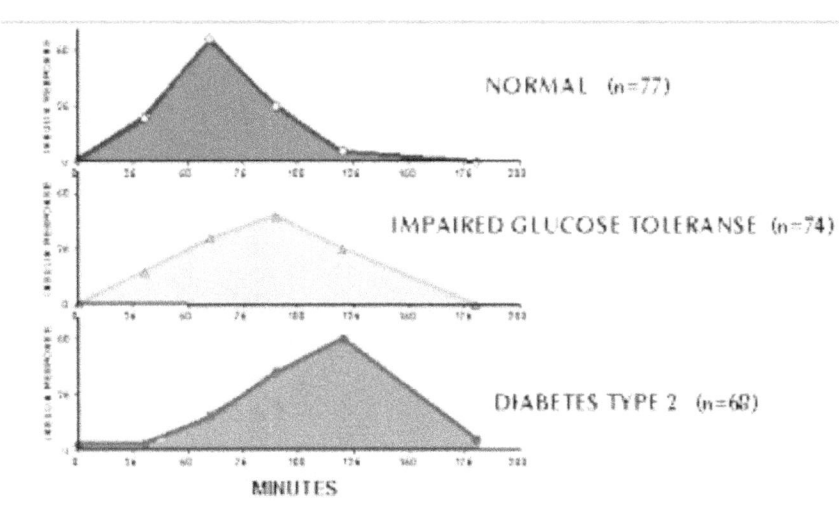

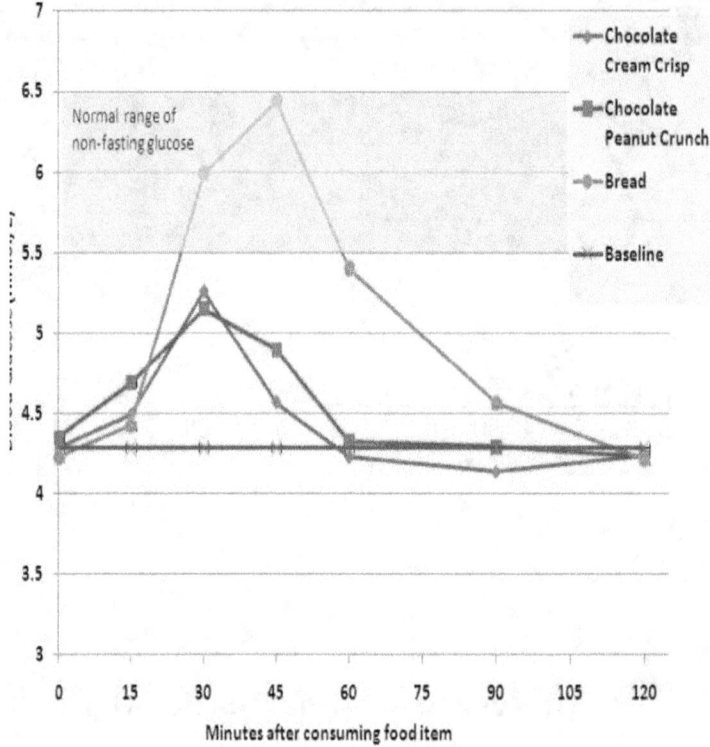

Plasma Glucose Levels After Consuming Isalean Bars or White Bread n = 13 subjects

Chapter 9: Classification of Carbohydrates

* * * * *

The term *Carbohydrate* comes from its Chemical nature. Carbohydrates contain the elements Carbon, Hydrogen, and Oxygen, with the Hydrogen/Oxygen ratio usually that of water (CH_2O).

Carbohydrates are classified according to the number of basic Sugar or Saccharide units that make up their structure.

The Monosaccharides and Disaccharides are referred to as *Simple Carbohydrates* because of their relatively small size and structure.

The Polysaccharides, including Starch and certain Fibers, are called *Complex Carbohydrates* based on their larger size and more complicated structure.

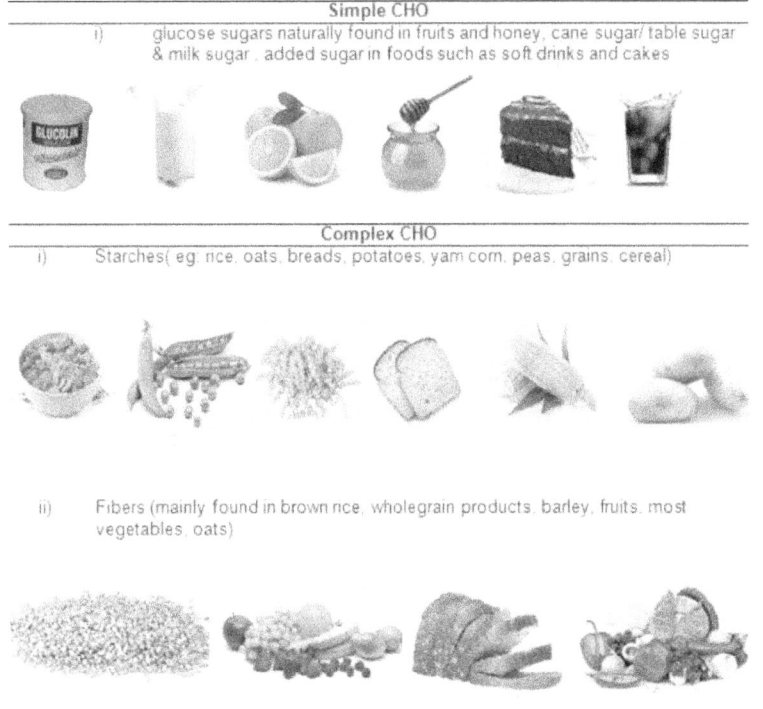

Simple CHO					
i)	glucose sugars naturally found in fruits and honey, cane sugar/ table sugar & milk sugar , added sugar in foods such as soft drinks and cakes				

Complex CHO				
i)	Starches(eg: rice, oats, breads, potatoes, yam corn, peas, grains, cereal)			

ii)   Fibers (mainly found in brown rice, wholegrain products, barley, fruits, most vegetables, oats)

Monosaccharides

Monosaccharides normally found in food

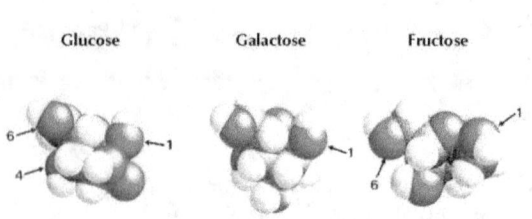

Glucose   Galactose   Fructose

The simplest form of a Carbohydrate is the **Monosaccharide**, or Single Sugar. The three Monosaccharides important in our Nutrition are (1) Glucose, (2) Fructose, and (3) Galactose. **Or Simple Carbohydrates**

Monosaccharides and Disaccharides are what we commonly refer to as *Sugars*.

Glucose, Fructose, and Galactose, each contains **6 Carbon, 12 Hydrogen,** and **6 Oxygen Atoms** ($C_6H_{12}O_6$), with the difference coming in their respective arrangements of these Atoms. Glucose, often called *Blood Sugar*, is the most important carbohydrate fuel for the human body.

Glucose

Glucose is a moderately sweet sugar found naturally in only a few foods, one being corn syrup.

a. Glucose, fructose, and galactose are monosaccharides that have the same chemical formulas, but the atoms are arranged differently.

Glucose is the common Body fuel that's Oxidized by our Cells.

It is supplied to the Body directly from the digestion of Starch, but it can also be obtained through the conversion of other Simple Sugars.

Glucose (referred to by its older name *Dextrose* in hospital intravenous solutions) is the form in which Carbohydrates circulate in our Blood which makes it and essential element to our Growth and development.

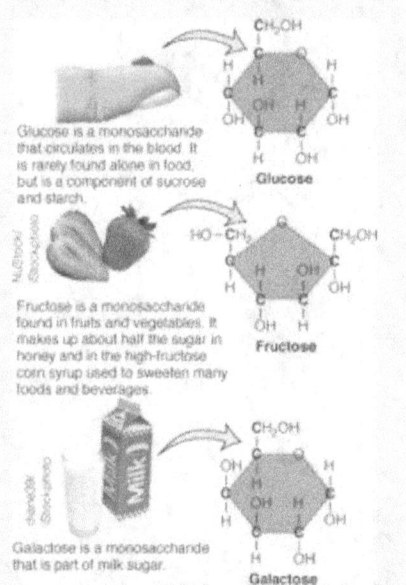

Glucose is a monosaccharide that circulates in the blood. It is rarely found alone in food, but is a component of sucrose and starch.

Glucose

Fructose is a monosaccharide found in fruits and vegetables. It makes up about half the sugar in honey and in the high-fructose corn syrup used to sweeten many foods and beverages.

Fructose

Galactose is a monosaccharide that is part of milk sugar.

Galactose

Fructose

Fructose is the sweetest of the Simple Sugars and is naturally found and abundant in Fruits and Honey.

Fructose intake has increased dramatically since the manufacturing of *High-Fructose Corn Syrup* (HFCS), which was introduced for use in processed food-like items.

HFCS is chemical used in many soft drinks, fruit drinks, commercial baked products, and dessert mixes to make them sweet.

Recent studies show that approximately 9% of the total Energy intake of Americans 2 years of age and older comes from manufactured and processed Fructose.

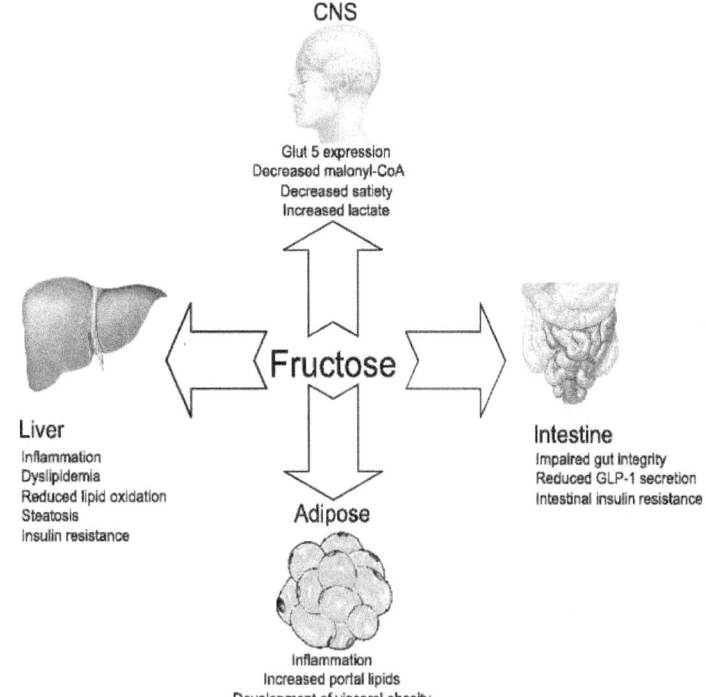

CNS
Glut 5 expression
Decreased malonyl-CoA
Decreased satiety
Increased lactate

Liver
Inflammation
Dyslipidemia
Reduced lipid oxidation
Steatosis
Insulin resistance

Intestine
Impaired gut integrity
Reduced GLP-1 secretion
Intestinal insulin resistance

Adipose
Inflammation
Increased portal lipids
Development of visceral obesity
Decreased lipoprotein clearance

In our Bodies Fructose is converted to Glucose and burned for Energy.

Fructose is absorbed less efficiently than Glucose, and amounts of approximately 25 to 50 grams or more leads to the cause of Gastrointestinal distress. For perspective, a 498-oz container of apple juice may contain 16 grams of Fructose, whereas a 12-oz can of a sweetened soft drink may supply 22 grams or more.

Galactose

The Simple Sugar Galactose is never found free in foods but is released in the digestion of Lactose (Milk Sugar) and its then converted to Glucose in our Liver. This reaction is reversible; during Lactation, Glucose is reconverted to Galactose for use in milk production.

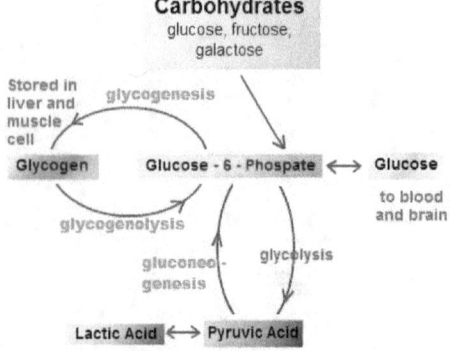

Nutrition In-Sight

1. Glucose, Fructose, and Galactose are Monosaccharides that have the same chemical formulas, but the Atoms are arranged in a different order.

2. Maltose, Sucrose, and Lactose are Disaccharides made up of different pairs of Monosaccharides.

3. Glycogen, Starches, and the Fiber Cellulose are Polysaccharides made up of straight or branching chains of Glucose.

PHYSIOLOGIC AND NUTRITIONAL SIGNIFICANCE OF MONOSACCHARIDES

MONOSACCHARIDE	SOURCE	SIGNIFICANCE
d-Glucose[*]	Fruit juices; hydrolysis of starch, cane sugar, maltose, and lactose	Form of sugar used by the body for fuel; found in blood and tissue fluids
d-Fructose	Fruit and fruit juices; honey; hydrolysis of sucrose from cane sugar	Converted to glucose in the liver and intestine to serve as body fuel
d-Galactose	Hydrolysis of lactose (milk sugar)	Converted to glucose in the liver to be used as body fuel; synthesized in the mammary gland to form lactose for milk; constituent of glycolipids and glycoproteins

[*]Monosaccharides can exist in d or l forms depending on the position of the hydroxyl group on the right (d) or left (l) side of a specific carbon. Digestive enzymes are stereospecific and act only on d sugars.

Disaccharides

The **Disaccharides** are Double Sugars, comprised of two Monosaccharides bonded together. There are three Disaccharides of physiologic importance to us - Sucrose, Lactose, and Maltose. Their Monosaccharide components are as follows:

b. Maltose, sucrose, and lactose are disaccharides made up of different pairs of monosaccharides.

Sucrose = 1 Glucose + 1 Fructose

Lactose = 1 Glucose + 1 Galactose

Maltose = 1 Glucose + 1 Glucose

Notice that Glucose is found in each of the Disaccharides.

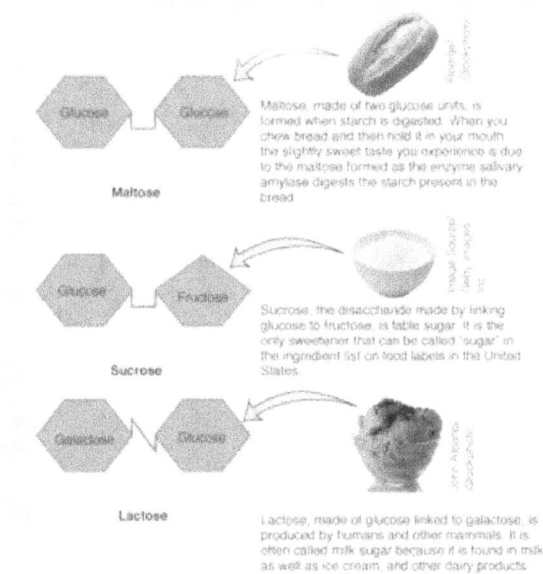

Maltose, made of two glucose units, is formed when starch is digested. When you chew bread and then hold it in your mouth the slightly sweet taste you experience is due to the maltose formed as the enzyme salivary amylase digests the starch present in the bread.

Sucrose, the disaccharide made by linking glucose to fructose, is table sugar. It is the only sweetener that can be called "sugar" in the ingredient list on food labels in the United States.

Lactose, made of glucose linked to galactose, is produced by humans and other mammals. It is often called milk sugar because it is found in milk as well as ice cream, and other dairy products.

Sucrose

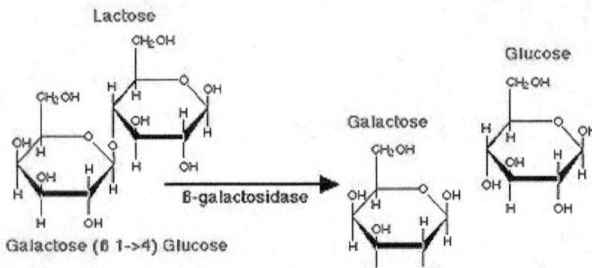

Sucrose is what is known as common "table sugar" and is made commercially from Sugar Cane and Sugar Beets.

It is found naturally in Molasses and certain Fruits and Vegetables (e.g., peaches and carrots) and is also added to almost all manufactured and processed foods.

Lactose

Lactose is the Sugar found in Milk and is the least sweet of the Disaccharides, with it being only about 1/6 as sweet as Sucrose. Even though Milk is relatively high in Lactose, its by-product cheese, may contain little or no Lactose depending on how the cheese is made. When Milk sours in the initial stage of cheese making, the liquid Whey separates from the solid curd. The Lactose from the Milk dissolves into the Whey, which is drained away and discarded. The remaining curd is processed into cheese, which makes it possible for many Lactose intolerant individuals to digest cheese, although particular cheeses vary in Lactose content.

Maltose

Maltose occurs naturally in relatively few foods but is formed in our bodies as an intermediate product in Starch digestion. It is found in commercial malt products and germinating cereal grains.

PHYSIOLOGIC AND NUTRITIONAL SIGNIFICANCE OF DISACCHARIDES

DISACCHARIDE	SOURCE	SIGNIFICANCE
Sucrose	Cane and beet sugar, sorghum cane, carrots, pineapple	Hydrolyzed to glucose and fructose; fuel for cells

DISACCHARIDE	SOURCE	SIGNIFICANCE
Lactose	Milk	Hydrolyzed to glucose and galactose; fuel for cells; milk production in lactation
Maltose	Starch digestion by Amylase or commercial hydrolysis; malt and germinating cereals	Hydrolyzed to yield two molecules of glucose; fuel for cells; can be fermented

Although Sugars occur naturally in Fruit and Milk, the major portion of Sugar in the U.S. diet is added in food preparation or processing. We add sugar when we pour syrup on pancakes or use table sugar to sweeten coffee, tea, or cereal. Various forms of sugar are added to pies, cakes, cookies, candy, soft drinks, fruit drinks, and breakfast cereals.

The average daily intake of added sugars in the United States is about 18 tsp (77 grams), nearly 15% of our total Energy intake.

Soda is the highest contributor to the added sugar intakes of most adults, and fruit drinks contribute most to the added Sugar intakes of children ages 2 to 5.

Although the consumption of added sugar fell by nearly 25% over the past decade, it still remains above the 2010 *Dietary Guidelines for Americans* recommendation of 8 tsp or less on a 2000 kcal diet.

Complex Carbohydrates are Polysaccharides and they are generally not sweet tasting the way Simple Carbs are. Theses Complex Carbs include **Glycogen** in animals and Starches and Fibers in Plants.

c. Glycogen, starches, and the fiber cellulose are polysaccharides made up of straight or branching chains of glucose.

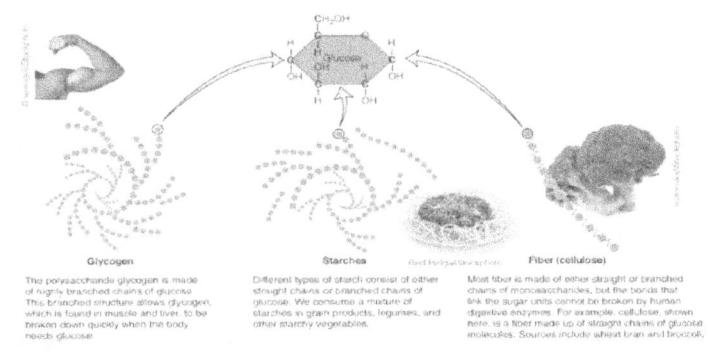

Glycogen	Starches	Fiber (cellulose)
The polysaccharide glycogen is made of highly branched chains of glucose. This branched structure allows glycogen, which is found in muscle and liver, to be broken down quickly when the body needs glucose.	Different types of starch consist of either straight chains or branched chains of glucose. We consume a mixture of starches in grain products, legumes, and other starchy vegetables.	Most fiber is made of either straight or branched chains of monosaccharides, but the bonds that link the sugar units cannot be broken by human digestive enzymes. For example, cellulose, shown here, is a fiber made up of straight chains of glucose molecules. Sources include wheat bran and broccoli.

Glycogen is the storage form of Glucose in us and other animals. It is found in our Liver and Muscles, but we don't consume it in our diet because soon after being slaughtered the Glycogen in animal muscles is broken down.

Glycogen is the storage form of Carbohydrates found in animals and is composed of many Glucose Molecules bonded together in a highly branched structure.

Polysaccharides

Complex Carbs are called *Polysaccharides* because they are made up of many (*Poly*) single Glucose (Saccharide) units. Starch is the most important digestible Polysaccharide and others are **Glycogen** and **Dextrin**. Non-digestible Polysaccharides, such as Cellulose, add important bulk to the diet and are categorized as **Dietary Fiber**.

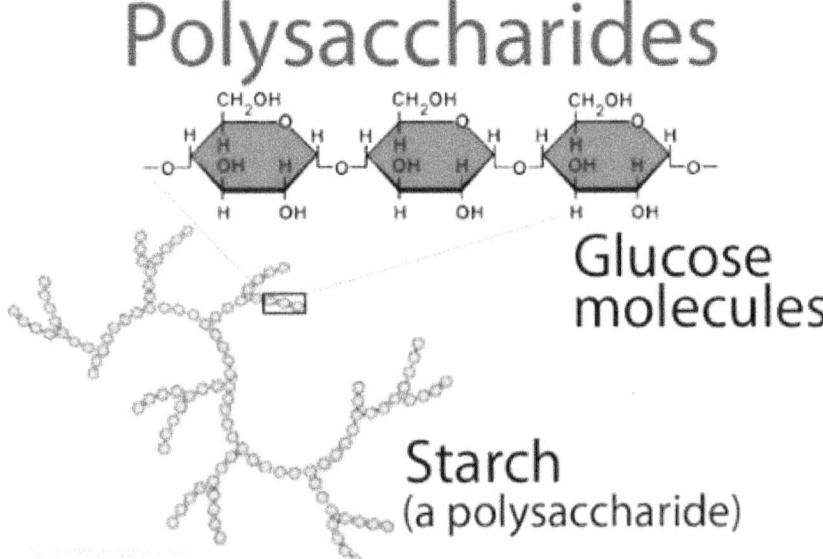

Chapter 10: Starch – Polysaccharide

* * * * *

Starch is made up of Glucose Molecules that are bonded together in either Straight or Branched Chains. It serves primarily as the Storage form of Carbohydrates in Plants and provides the Energy that Plants need and utilize for growth and reproduction. Consequently, when we eat these Plants – Fruits and Veggies, we consume this Stored Energy and our Bodies use it just like the Plants = Growth and Reproduction!!

One of the main forms that this Energy is manifested is in the form of Starch.

The word "Starch" is from a Germanic root with the meanings "strong, stiff, strengthen, stiffen". The modern German word - Stärke (Starch) is closely related.

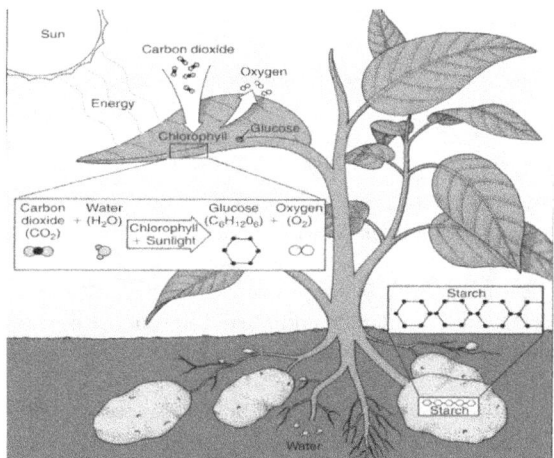

FIGURE 3-1   Photosynthesis. In the presence of sunlight and the green leaf pigment chlorophyll, plants use water and carbon dioxide (CO_2) to produce glucose and starch by capturing the sun's energy and transforming it into chemical energy in the food products stored in their roots, stems, and leaves; through this process oxygen is returned to the atmosphere. (Courtesy Medical and Scientific Illustration.)

The word "Amylum" for Starch has its root in the Greek αμυλον, "Amylon" which means "not ground at a mill". The root word 'Amyl' is used in Biochemistry for several of the compounds that are related to Starch.

Amylum is a Polymeric Carbohydrate that consists of a large number of Glucose units joined by Glycosidic Bonds.

This manifestation of Polysaccharide is produced by most Green Plants. The best sources of these Green color based Plants is in the form of Sea Veggies (Sea Weed, Spirulina).

Starch is the most common Carbohydrate present in our diets, mainly in the form of staple foods like potatoes, wheat, maize or corn, rice and cassava as the biggest contributors.

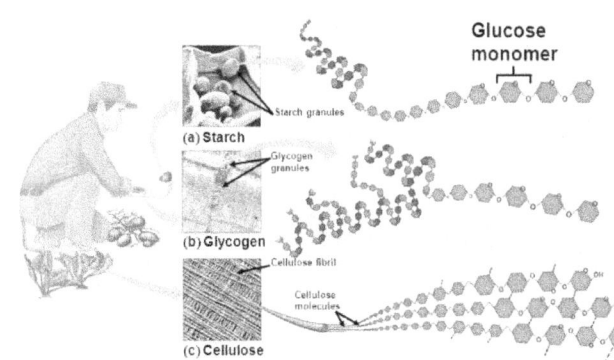

Properties of starch raw material

	Appearance/ Texture	Flavour	Clarity
Potato	pulpy	no	transparent
Maize	smooth slightly gellified	cereal	opaque
Waxy maize	smooth	cereal	opaque
Tapioca	very smooth	no	transparent
Wheat	smooth slightly gellified	cereal	opaque
Barley AP	very smooth	cereal	opaque

Pure Starch presents in a white, tasteless and odorless powder form that is insoluble in cold water or alcohol.

Starch consists of two types of Molecules: a Linear and Helical Amylose and then a Branched Amylopectin.

Depending on the Plant, the amount of Starch generally contains approximately 20 to 25% Amylose with an approximate 75 to 80% of Amylopectin by weight. Glycogen, which is the Glucose store of humans and animals, is more of a branched version of the element Amylopectin.

Our Digestive Enzymes have problems Digesting the Crystalline structures and Raw Starch will digest poorly in our Duodenum and Small Intestine. However, some Bacterial degradation will take place mainly in the Colon. When starch is cooked, the digestibility of it is increased.

Starch consists of many coiled and branching chains of Single Glucose units and will yield only Glucose at the completion of Digestion. Cooking Starch will not only improve the flavor of Starch but the cooking process also softens and ruptures the Starch Cells which makes Digestion easier.

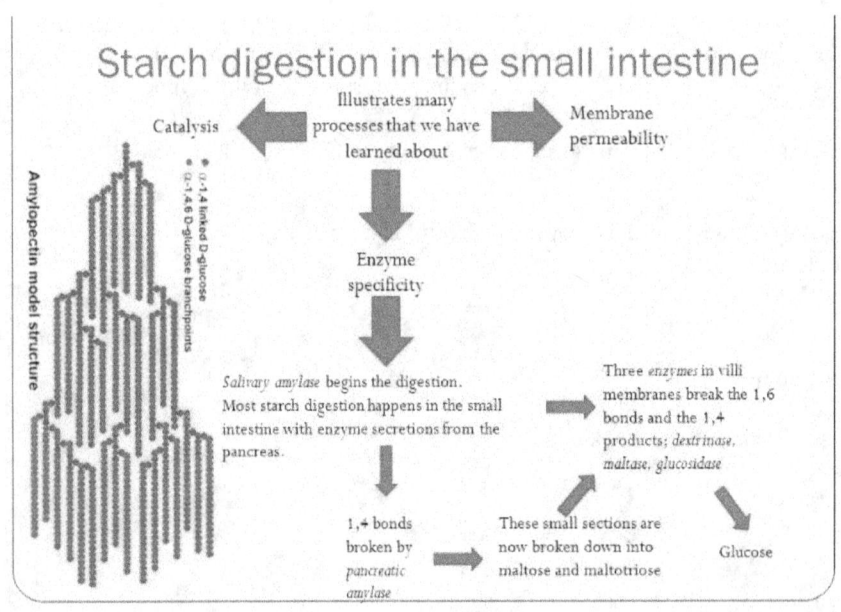

Starch digestion in the small intestine

STARCH AND ENERGY

Historically, people consumed large amounts of uncooked and unprocessed starch-containing plants, which contained high amounts of resistant starch. Microbes within the large intestine fermented the starch, produced short-chain fatty acids, which were used as energy as well as maintenance and growth of the microbes.

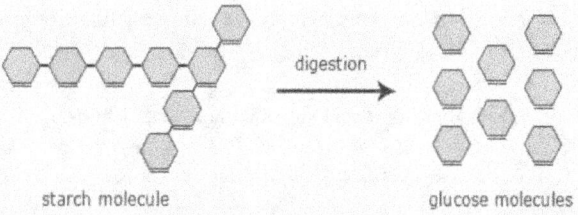

Starches, as well as Sugars, eventually break-down into Glucose -- our body's main LIFE Fuel source.

When we chew, the Saliva in your mouth begins deconstructing Starch into smaller Molecules of Carbs that are called Maltose. Once these new formed Maltose Molecules reach our gut, the Digestive juices further break them down into Glucose. The Villi that line our Intestinal walls pick up these Glucose Molecules and absorb them directly into our Bloodstream.

Since the digestion of Starches has several steps, naturally occurring Starches slowly elevate our Blood Sugar levels and keep our Blood Sugar stable for a while before it drops again. We don't suffer the Effect from a sudden DROP of Energy as Caused by artificial Starches in comparison, with Naturally occurring Starch, we experience the Effect of extended Energy.

The amounts of the various elements of Nutrition that we need is measured in Grams (g) and/or Milligrams (mg). These are NOT large amounts. But the wonderful thing is that Naturally occurring Nutrients pack a POWERFUL Punch in small packages (amounts)!!!!!

Better choices of our dietary Starch intake allows us to eat less which significantly decreases the wear and tear on the Engine of our Body = STOMACH. Our Immune System is manifested from within our Digestive system which makes our food choices literally our Death or our LIFE !!

There are two types of Polysaccharides that our Body uses for storing Energy: Starch and Glycogen. These naturally occurring Starches serve as our short-term Energy stores and are made from a mixture of Amylose and Amylopectin.

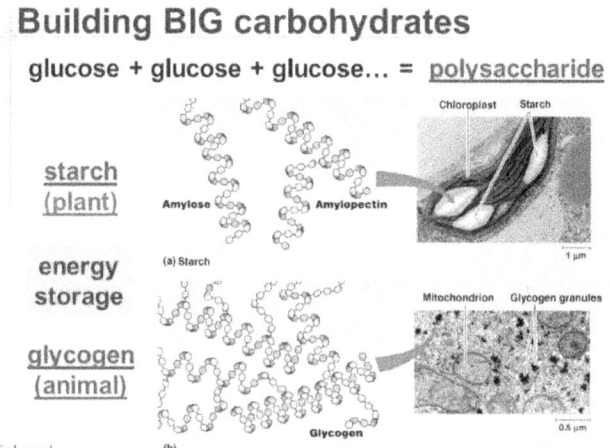

Some of the common dietary Starches include rice, potatoes, wheat, and corn. The element Glycogen, on the other hand, acts as a long-term storage option. Glycogen is mainly produced by our Liver and Muscles, but it can also be made during the process called Glycogenesis, which occurs in both our Brain and Stomach.

Understanding both the direct and supporting role that Starches play in our health and fitness makes the quality we choose even more vital. Manufactured or processed Starches are DEVOID of the Life Energy from the Sun, so they don't support any of the above mentioned Body functions or organs. In fact, when consumed their material becomes TOXIC and the Energy released is empty and negative.

Good vs. Bad Carbohydrates

Complex Sugars	vs.	Simple Sugars
Low GI	vs.	High GI
High Quality	vs.	Low Quality
Unrefined	vs.	Refined

Whole Foods vs. Processed Foods

The Role of Starch /Polysaccharides in Nutrition

Polysaccharides are critical when it comes to proper nutrition because they comprise the Complex Carbohydrates that, for serves as our body's primary LIFE Energy source. Every one of our Bodily functions relies on Carbohydrates for the supply of LIFE Energy. And while our bodies do have the ability where it can produce some Energy, it's certainly not enough to sustain itself. So we have to Eat the best forms of LIFE Energy present.

If we don't take in enough Carbs, we will have to instead supplement our LIFE Energy from other secondary sources that aren't as proficiently as Carbs. When you don't get enough Carbohydrates, the body is placed in immediate risk for physical symptoms. Examples of these symptoms include a drop in blood sugar, and feelings of weakness, and lightheadedness.

Polysaccharides does help us overcome fatigue, support healthy blood pressure and blood sugar, encourage a positive mood, soothe irritation, support Immune function, promote Cardiovascular health and even increase Libido.

Starches are Complex Carbs that require an extended period of time to break down. We should think of Starch as our time-release type of LIFE Energy. When you consume naturally occurring Starchy foods, you'll have a sustained Energy level over a period of several hours. This is different from the naturally occurring Sugars, which are Simple Carbohydrates that provides us with a quick surge of Energy, but does little to nothing to keep your Energy levels going. Which is the Primary function and addition of these dietary Starches.

Because the Glucose from Carbohydrates is essential to fuel every one of our Cells, most of our KCalories should come from Carbs. Both starches and naturally occurring Sugars, from Dairy, Fruits and Veggies should and must contribute to our overall balanced Carbohydrate intake.

Your diet should consist of approximately 45 to 65% Carbohydrates, which have 4 calories per gram, says the Dietary Guidelines for Americans 2010.

For an example, if you are following a 2,200-calorie daily diet, it means you need 247 to

Health Benefits of Fiber (non-starch polysaccharides)

1. Normalizes transit time of transport of food through the digestive track
2. Decreases serum cholesterol
3. Slows food absorption which decreases peak serum glucose levels
4. Binds bile acids, some of which are carcinogens
5. Dilutes gut contents which can protect against toxic materials
6. Increases "healthful" bacteria and reduced ph of the intestinal tract
7. Increases production of short chain fatty acids which are beneficial to the intestinal mucosa   28

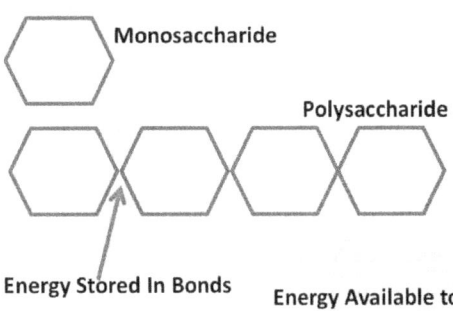

Monosaccharide

Polysaccharide

Energy Stored In Bonds

Energy Available to Cells When Bonds Broken!

357 total grams of naturally occurring Carbs each day to sustain your Energy levels and fuel your body.

STARCH USES IN FOOD

- Anti-crystallising in **confectioneries**;
- Sweetening power in **beverages**;
- Bulking agent / texture in **dairy** products;
- Preservatives in **jams**;
- Moistening in **bakery products**;
- Freezing point depression in **ice creams**;
- Thickening, binding agent in **soups & sauces**;
- Browning effect in **caramels**;
- Cooling effect in **chewing-gum**;
- Low glycemic index in **dietetic food**...

Whole foods that are minimally processed and naturally high in Starch are also often low on the Glycemic Index. The Glycemic Index scale, or GI for short, ranks foods from 1 to 100, depending on how quickly they raise our Blood Sugar. Foods that are low on the Glycemic Index have a rating of 55 or below and include Starchy foods like Whole-Grain bread, oatmeal, brown rice, all varieties of beans, yams and peas. Since these foods slowly elevate our Blood Sugar levels, they create the effect that allows us to be Energized all afternoon.

As foods became and continues to become more processed, they are made more easily digested as well as being able to release more Glucose in the Small Intestine, which results in less Starch reaching the Large Intestine and more Energy being absorbed by the Human body.

This Un-Natural shift in our Energy delivery is a leading contributing factor to the development of Metabolic disorders of modern life, including OBESITY and DIABETES.

The refining process and manufacturing procedures used by food companies strips these naturally occurring Starches and removes their Natural Life Energy properties and literally leaving just a carcass – DEVOID OF THE SUN!!!

Resistant Starch is a form of Starch that isn't digested in our Small Intestine. Amylose Starch from corn has a higher Gelatinization temperature than other types of starch and retains its Resistant Starch properties through baking, mild extrusion and other food processing techniques.

Type of Resistant Starch	Description	Examples
RS1	Physically inaccessible, non-digestible matrix	Whole or partly milled grains and seeds
RS2	Tightly packed, ungelatinized starch granules	Raw potato starch Green bananas High-amylose cornstarch
RS3	Retrograded starch (cooled gelatinized starch)	Cooked and cooled potato, bread and pudding
RS4	Chemically modified starch	Etherized, esterified or cross-bonded starches (used in processed foods)

It is usually used as an Insoluble dietary Fiber in processed foods such as bread, pasta, cookies, crackers, pretzels and other low moisture foods.

The types of this Resistant Starch that these companies use is what makes their food-like products TOXIC inside the Human Body.

In some forms it is also utilized as a dietary supplement for its health benefits. Published studies have shown that naturally occurring forms of Resistant Starch helps to improve Insulin sensitivity, increases satiety and improves markers of Colonic function. We must always remember that these health benefits of Resistant Starch id from intact Whole Grains.

Applications of Modified Starch Products

Sauces(Mayonnaise)
- Water binding capacity
- Thickening
- stabilization

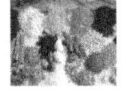

Beverages (Tea, coffee)
- Stable emulsions
- Good dispersibility
- High solubility
- Low viscosity

As an additive used for food processing, food Starches are typically used as thickeners and stabilizers in foods such as puddings, custards, soups, sauces, gravies, pie fillings, and salad dressings, and to make noodles and pastas, extenders, emulsion stabilizers and are exceptional binders in processed meats.

Starch mixtures thicken when cooked because the element encasing the Starch Granules has a gel-like quality that thickens mixtures in the same way as Pectin causes jelly to set. Dissolving starch in warm water forms a Wheat-paste, which is then used as a thickening, stiffening or gluing agent.

Starch becomes Soluble in Water when heated. The Granules swell and burst, the semi-crystalline structure is lost and the smaller Amylose Molecules start leaching out of the Granule, and begins forming a network that holds Water and increasing the mixture's viscosity. This process is called starch Gelatinization.

During cooking, Starch becomes a paste and increases further in Viscosity. During cooling or prolonged storage of the paste, this semi-crystalline structure partially recovers and the Starch paste starts to thicken, expelling Water in the process. This reaction is mainly caused by Retro-gradation of the Amylose. This process what is responsible for the hardening of bread or making it stale, and for Synersis which is the Water layer on top of a Starch-gel.

Gummed sweets such as jelly beans and wine gums are not manufactured using a mold in the conventional sense. A tray is filled with native Starch and leveled. A positive mold is then pressed into the starch leaving an impression of 1,000 or so jelly beans. The jelly mix is then poured into the impressions and put into a stove to set. This method greatly reduces the number of molds that must be manufactured.

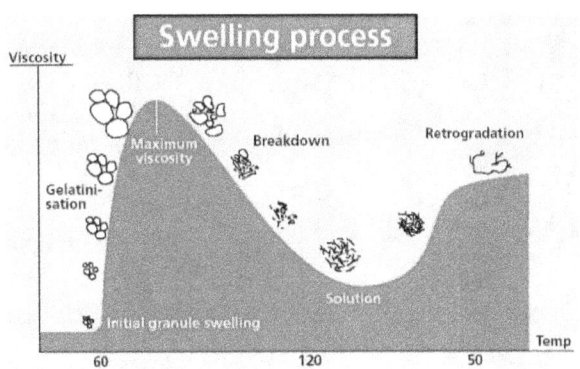

The Starch Industry

The Starch industry extracts and refines Starches from Seeds, Roots and Tubers, through procedures of wet grinding, washing, sieving and drying. Today, the main commercial refined Starches are derived from Cornstarch, Tapioca, Wheat, Rice and Potato Starch. To a lesser extent other sources include Rice, Sweet Potato, Sago and Mung Bean. From a historical perspective, Florida Arrowroot has also become commercialized and at the time of this writing, Starch is extracted from more than 50 types of Plants.

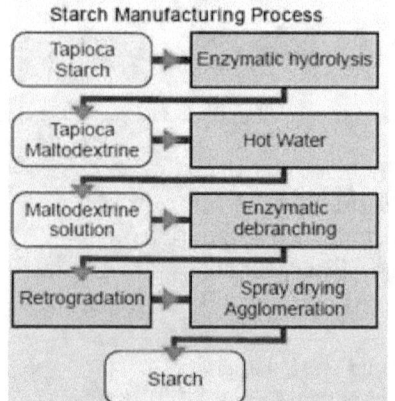

Starch Manufacturing Process

Untreated Starch requires heat to thicken or gelatinize. When a Starch is pre-cooked, it can then be used to thicken instantly in cold water and this chemical reaction makes what is referred to as a Pre-Gelatinized Starch.

In the food manufacturing and processing industry, Starch is converted into Sugars and this is usually accomplished by malting, and fermenting to produce Ethanol in the manufacture of beer, whisky and bio-fuels. It is also processed to produce many of the TOXIC Sugars that are used in almost all processed and manufactured food-like products.

Almost every Green Plant uses Starch as their Energy store. An exception is the family Asteraceae (Asters, Daisies and Sunflowers), where Starch is replaced in these Plants by the element Fructan Inulin.

In Photosynthesis, Plants uses the Un-Seen LIFE Energy from the Sun to produce the Seen Chemical Glucose with the addition of our Carbon Dioxide. This Glucose is used in one of 2 ways: to make the Cellulose Fibers, which are the structural components of the Plant; or it is stored in the form of Starch Granules, in Amyloplasts.

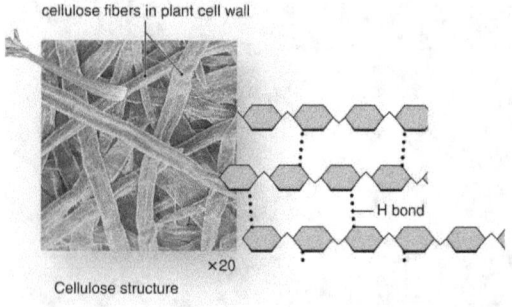

cellulose fibers in plant cell wall

×20

Cellulose structure

Toward the end of the growing season, this Starch accumulates in twigs of Trees near the Buds. Fruit, seeds, rhizomes, and tubers begin to store their Starch to prepare for the next growing season.

Normally Glucose is Soluble in Water, Hydrophilic, and binds with Water which then takes up much of the Plants space and is also Osmotically Active.

Glucose that manifests in the form of Starch, on the other hand, is not Soluble, therefore it is Osmotically Inactive and can be stored in a much more compact fashion making this form more abundant.

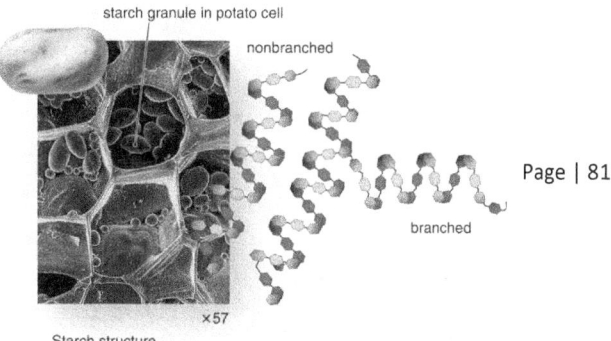

Glucose molecules are bound in Starch by the easily formed Hydrolyzed Alpha Bonds. This is the same type of Bond that is found in the animal reserve Polysaccharide Glycogen. This is in contrast to many structural Polysaccharides such as Chitin, Cellulose and Peptidoglycan, which are bound by Beta Bonds and are much more resistant to Hydrolysis.

Starch is synthesized in Plant leaves during the day, in order to serve as an Energy source at night. Starch is stored as granules and the Molecules arrange themselves in the Plant in semi-crystalline granules. Each plant species has a unique starch granular size: rice starch is relatively small (about 2µm) while potato starches have larger granules (up to 100µm).

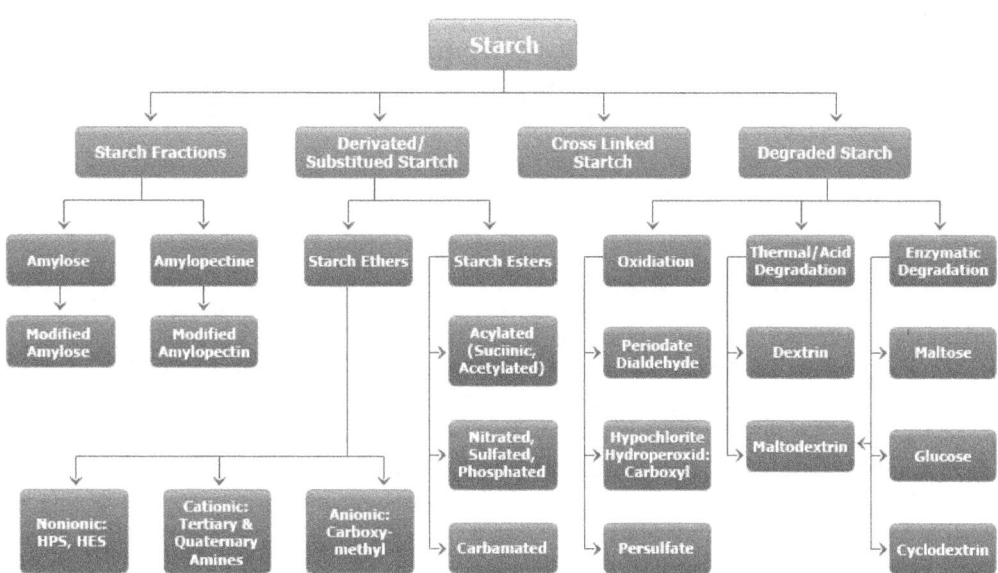

Starch Sugars

Starch can be Hydrolyzed into simpler Carbohydrates through reactions caused by Acids, various Enzymes, or a combination of the two. The resulting fragments are known as Dextrins. The extent of conversion is typically quantified by Dextrose Equivalent (DE), which is roughly the fraction of the Glycosidic Bonds in Starch that have been broken.

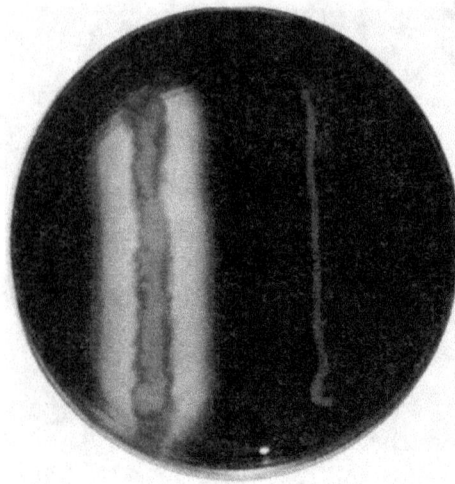

Starch

Clear zone along left streak indicates starch hydrolysis.

These Starch Sugars are by far the most common starch based food ingredient and are used as sweetener in many drinks and foods and they are the most TOXIC.........Completely DEVOID of the Sun.

They include:

Maltodextrin: a lightly Hydrolyzed (DE 10–20) Starch product used as a bland-tasting filler and thickener. *This by-product is TOXIC if consumed!*

Various Glucose syrups (DE 30–70), also called Corn Syrups here in the US. Its Viscous solutions are used as sweeteners and thickeners in many kinds of processed foods. *These by-products are TOXIC if consumed!*

Dextrose (DE 100), a commercial Glucose that is prepared by the complete Hydrolysis of Starch. *This by-product is TOXIC if consumed!*

High Fructose Corn Syrup: this TOXIC product is made by treating Dextrose solutions with the Enzyme Glucose Isomerase, until a substantial fraction of the Glucose has been UN-Naturally converted into Fructose. In the United States sugar prices are two to three times higher than in the rest of the world, which makes High Fructose Corn Syrup significantly cheaper, and has fast become the principal sweetener used in processed foods and beverages. One kind of High Fructose Corn Syrup, HFCS-55, is sweeter than sucrose because it is made with more Fructose, while the sweetness of HFCS-42 is on par with Sucrose.

This by-product is TOXIC if consumed!

Sugar Alcohols, such as Maltitol, Erythritol, Sorbitol, Mannitol and Hydrogenated Starch Hydrolysate, are TOXIC sweeteners made by reducing sugars.

Modified starches

A Modified Starch is a Starch that has been Chemically Modified to allow the Starch to function properly under conditions frequently encountered during processing or storage, such as high heat, high shear, low pH, freeze/thaw and cooling.

The modified food starches are E coded according to the International Numbering System for Food Additives (INS):

1400 Dextrin

1401 Acid-treated starch

1402 Alkaline-treated starch

1403 Bleached starch

1404 Oxidized starch

1405 Starches, enzyme-treated

1410 Monostarch phosphate

1412 Distarch phosphate

1413 Phosphated distarch phosphate

1414 Acetylated distarch phosphate

1420 Starch acetate

1422 Acetylated distarch adipate

1440 Hydroxypropyl starch

1442 Hydroxypropyl distarch phosphate

1443 Hydroxypropyl distarch glycerol

1450 Starch sodium octenyl succinate

1451 Acetylated oxidized starch

INS 1400, 1401, 1402, 1403 and 1405 are in the EU food ingredients without an E-number. Typical modified starches for technical applications are cationic starches, hydroxyethyl starch and carboxymethylated starches.

Starch Industrial Applications

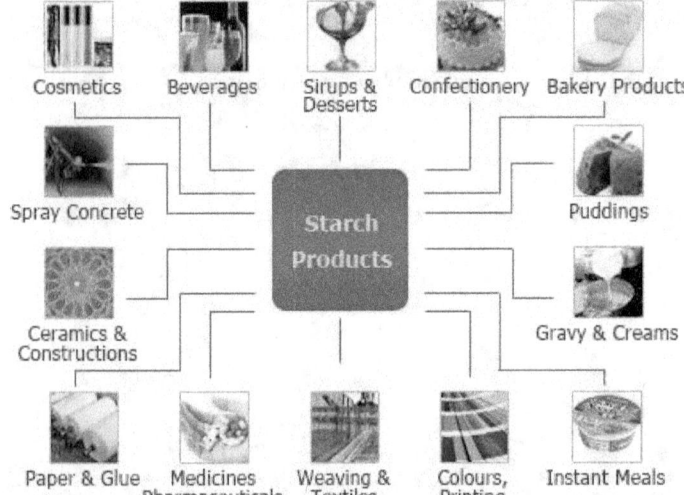

Papermaking

Papermaking is the largest non-food application for Starches globally, consuming millions of metric tons annually.

In a typical sheet of copy paper for instance, the Starch content may be as high as 8%.

Both chemically modified and unmodified Starches are used in papermaking.

In the wet part of the papermaking process, generally called the "wet-end", the starches used are cationic and have a positive charge bound to the starch polymer. These starch derivatives associate with the anionic or negatively charged paper fibers / cellulose and inorganic fillers.

Cationic Starches together with other retention and internal sizing agents help to give the necessary strength properties to the paper web formed in the papermaking process (wet strength), and to provide strength to the final paper sheet (dry strength).

In the dry end of the papermaking process, the paper web is rewetted with a starch based solution. The process is called surface sizing. Starches used have been chemically, or enzymatically depolymerized at the paper mill or by the starch industry (oxidized starch). The size/starch solutions are applied to the paper web by means of various mechanical presses (size presses).

Together with surface sizing agents the surface starches impart additional strength to the paper web and additionally provide water hold out or "size" for superior printing properties. Starch is also used in paper coatings as one of the binders for the coating formulations which include a mixture of pigments, binders and thickeners. Coated paper has improved smoothness, hardness, whiteness and gloss and thus improves printing characteristics.

Corrugated board adhesives

Corrugated board adhesives are the next largest application of non-food starches globally. Starch glues are mostly based on unmodified native starches, plus some additive such as borax and caustic soda. Part of the starch is gelatinized to carry the slurry of uncooked starches and prevent sedimentation. This opaque glue is called a Stein-Hall adhesive. The glue is applied on tips of the fluting. The fluted paper is pressed to paper called liner. This is then dried under high heat, which causes the rest of the uncooked starch in glue to swell/gelatinize. This gelatinizing makes the glue a fast and strong adhesive for corrugated board production.

Clothing starch

Clothing or laundry starch is a liquid that is prepared by mixing a vegetable starch in water (earlier preparations also had to be boiled), and is used in the laundering of clothes. Starch was widely used in Europe in the 16th and 17th centuries to stiffen the wide collars and ruffs of fine linen which surrounded the necks of the well-to-do. During the 19th century and early 20th century, it was stylish to stiffen the collars and sleeves of men's shirts and the ruffles of girls' petticoats by applying starch to them as the clean clothes were being ironed. Aside from the smooth, crisp edges it gave to clothing, it served practical purposes as well. Dirt and sweat from a person's neck and wrists would stick to the starch rather than to the fibers of the clothing, and would easily wash away along with the starch. After each laundering, the starch would be reapplied. Today, the product is sold in aerosol cans for home use.

Another large non-food starch application is in the construction industry, where starch is used in the gypsum wall board manufacturing process. Chemically modified or unmodified starches are added to the stucco containing primarily gypsum. Top and bottom heavyweight sheets of paper are applied to the formulation, and the process is allowed to heat and cure to form the eventual rigid wall board. The starches act as a glue for the cured gypsum rock with the paper covering, and also provide rigidity to the board.

Starch is used in the manufacture of various adhesives or glues[40] for book-binding, wallpaper adhesives, paper sack production, tube winding, gummed paper, envelope adhesives, school glues and bottle labeling. Starch derivatives, such as yellow dextrins, can be modified by addition of some chemicals to form a hard glue for paper work; some of those forms use borax or soda ash, which are mixed with the starch solution at 50–70 °C (122–158 °F) to create a very good adhesive. Sodium Silicate can be added to reinforce this formula.

Textile chemicals from starch: warp sizing agents are used to reduce breaking of yarns during weaving. Starch is mainly used to size cotton based yarns. Modified starch is also used as textile printing thickener.

In oil exploration, starch is used to adjust the viscosity of drilling fluid, which is used to lubricate the drill head and suspend the grinding residue in petroleum extraction.

Starch is also used to make some packing peanuts, and some drop ceiling tiles.

In the printing industry, food grade starch[41] is used in the manufacture of anti-set-off spray powder used to separate printed sheets of paper to avoid wet ink being set off.

For body powder, powdered corn starch is used as a substitute for talcum powder, and similarly in other health and beauty products.

Starch is used to produce various bioplastics, synthetic polymers that are biodegradable. An example is polylactic acid based on glucose from starch.

Glucose from starch can be further fermented to biofuel corn ethanol using the so-called wet milling process. Today most bioethanol production plants use the dry milling process to ferment corn or other feedstock directly to ethanol.

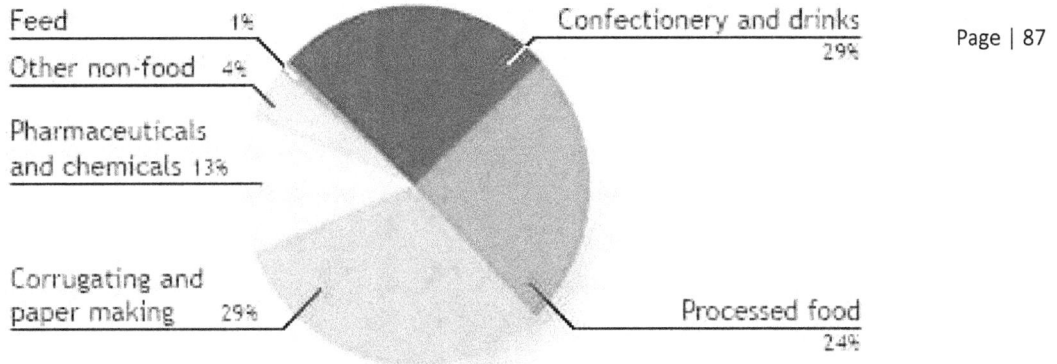

Feed 1%
Other non-food 4%
Pharmaceuticals and chemicals 13%
Corrugating and paper making 29%
Confectionery and drinks 29%
Processed food 24%

Total non-food applications : 47%   Total food applications : 53%

Chapter 11: Fiber: The Non-Digestible Carbohydrate

* * * * *

Fiber is basically the natural and non-digestible material found in Whole-Grain cereals, Fruits, Vegetables, and Legumes which is also commonly referred to as **Roughage.**

Due to the fact that our Digestive System lacks the necessary Enzymes necessary to break down these Complex Carbohydrates into forms that can be absorbed, they travel the length of the gastrointestinal tract and are eliminated in the feces.

Years of age	Grams of Fibre Per Day	
	Male	Female
1-2	19	19
4-8	25	25
9-13	31	26
14-18	38	26
19-50	38	25
> 50	30	21

The ability of Fiber to promote regular bowel function has been recognized for generations and long been a recognizable necessity.

All types of Fiber are beneficial to health, but of course, different Fibers have different Physiologic effects which makes knowing what type(s) of Fiber the food you eat contain even more important.

It also is the best way for us to successfully plan a meal that supplies various types. Making or preparing our own foods/meals is the best way to incorporate and ensure the quality and value of what you are eating.

Although most foods contain more than one type of Fiber, they likely have more of one than another so a little research maybe required to make the best choices and helps avoid over-loading on just one type.

Fiber is a type of Complex Carbohydrate that cannot be broken down by our Digestive Enzymes and therefore Fiber cannot be absorbed in our Small

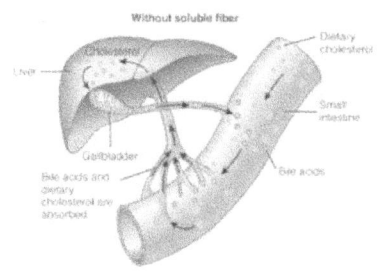

a. In the absence of soluble fiber, dietary cholesterol and bile, which contains cholesterol and bile acids made from cholesterol, are absorbed into the blood and transported to the liver for use in the body.

Intestine, and it passes straight through and into our Large Intestine. Along the way, this Fiber (depending on the type) gathers up bulk the is comprised of previously digested foods and helps push them along our Intestinal Tract and form into feces to be removed.

Soluble Fiber

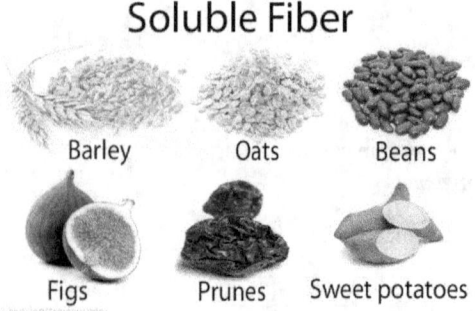

Barley   Oats   Beans

Figs   Prunes   Sweet potatoes

Fiber also includes several Chemical substances, some of which are soluble in Water.

Soluble fiber is found around the outside and inside of the Plant Cells and naturally dissolves in Water to form viscous solutions.

Although our Digestive Enzymes can't digest Soluble Fiber, we have Bacteria in our Large Intestine can metabolize it.

Legumes/Pulses/Beans contain this type of Soluble Fiber, in addition to small Polysaccharides, which are called **Oligosaccharides**, that also cannot be Metabolized by our Digestive Enzymes. Both of these pass into the Large Intestine, where they are Digested by Bacteria which is how flatulence or gas and other by-products are created. Examples of other foods that contain Soluble Fiber are Oats, Apples, and Seaweed.

Soluble Fiber dissolves in Water and/or absorbs Water and is readily broken down by our Intestinal Microflora. It also includes Pectins, Gums, and some Hemicelluloses.

Oligosaccharides are a manifestation of Carbohydrates that are comprised of approximately 3 to 10 Sugar units.

Fiber that does not dissolve in Water is called **Insoluble Fiber**. The primary source of Insoluble Fiber derives from the structural parts of Plants, such as Cell Walls.

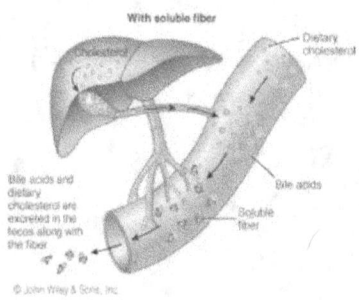

This is the type of Fiber that adds bulk to our Fecal matter because it passes in a relatively unchanged state through our Gastrointestinal Tract.

b. When soluble fiber is present in the digestive tract, the fiber binds cholesterol and bile acids so that they are excreted rather than absorbed. This helps reduce the amount of cholesterol in the body.

We need a regular and steady supply of Insoluble Fibers. They help to prevent the harmful build-up of bad bacteria from rotting or fermenting foods in our Intestinal Tracts.

Insoluble Fiber

Cereals   Whole-wheat bread   Lentils

To achieve maximum health and fitness we must ensure that we have as much matter leaving us as we are putting into ourselves.

Some examples of Food sources of Insoluble Fiber include Wheat and Rye Bran, Broccoli, and Celery.

Insoluble Fiber does not dissolve in Water and is less readily broken down by Bacteria in our large intestine.

Apple   Avocado   Strawberries

Manifestations of Insoluble Fiber includes Cellulose, some Hemicelluloses, and Lignin.

Research and studies of Fiber lead to the conclusion that the health benefits of Fiber are dependent on two characteristics: Viscosity and Fermentability. Viscous Fibers, which used to be referred to as *Soluble* Fibers, has a positive influence on our Blood Glucose levels and helps us to maintain and/or lower LDL-Cholesterol levels.

**Fibers that are fermented by the Microflora in our Gastrointestinal Tract and help provide bulk to and move our stools were referred to as *Insoluble* Fibers. However, we know that not all Viscous Fibers aren't Soluble, and not all Fibers that influence Laxation are Insoluble, which makes these terms no longer adequate or used to describe the health benefits of Fiber, BUT FOOD MANUFACTURES STILL USE THESE OUT-DATED TERMS TO CONFUSE AND MIS-LEAD ABOUT THEIR FOOD-LIKE PRODUCT.

Fiber is also used sometimes by these manufacturers to change the physical properties of food-like products. Pectin, a Soluble Fiber that's found in Fruits and Veggies, is added to jams and jellies as a thickener.

Gums are also used as thickeners because they have the ability to combine with water to keep solutions from separating.

Gum Arabic, Gum Karaya, Guar Gum, Locust Bean Gum, Xanthan Gum, and **Gum Tragacanth** are extracted from shrubs, trees, and seedpods; in addition to Agar, Carrageenan, and Alginates, which are Gums that are derived from Seaweed, are frequently added to these food-like products.

The health benefits of a high-Fiber diet has created consumer demand for high-Fiber foods.

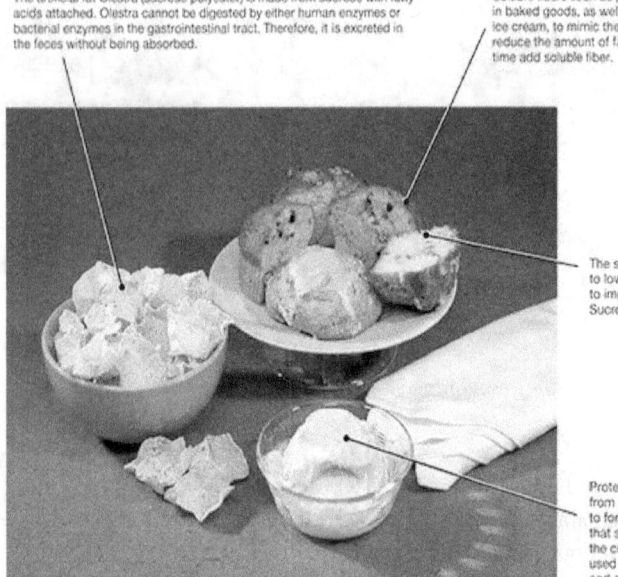

The artificial fat Olestra (sucrose polyester) is made from sucrose with fatty acids attached. Olestra cannot be digested by either human enzymes or bacterial enzymes in the gastrointestinal tract. Therefore, it is excreted in the feces without being absorbed.

Soluble fibers such as pectins and gums are often used in baked goods, as well as salad dressings, sauces, and ice cream, to mimic the texture that fat provides. They reduce the amount of fat in a product and at the same time add soluble fiber.

The sugar sucrose is usually added to low-fat and nonfat baked goods to improve flavor and add volume. Sucrose adds 4 Calories per gram.

Protein-based fat replacers are made from milk and egg proteins processed to form millions of microscopic balls that slide over each other, mimicking the creamy texture of fat.[43] They are used in frozen desserts, cheese foods, and other products but cannot be used for frying because they break down at high temperatures.

Wheat bran, which provides Insoluble Fiber, is a major element added to foods like breads and muffins to increase their Fiber content. But there has to be caution taken when consuming Wheat Bran because it is the part of the Wheat Grain that has little to no Nutritional value and only adds the Insoluble factor to our diets. The Bran is the outer protective casing.

A diet that's high in the consumption of Wheat Bran isn't an adequate source of Nutrition.

Fiber is added to food during processing for a variety of reasons, unfortunately the main reason is to replace the natural Fiber that was stripped away during the manufacturing/processing of making these food-like products.

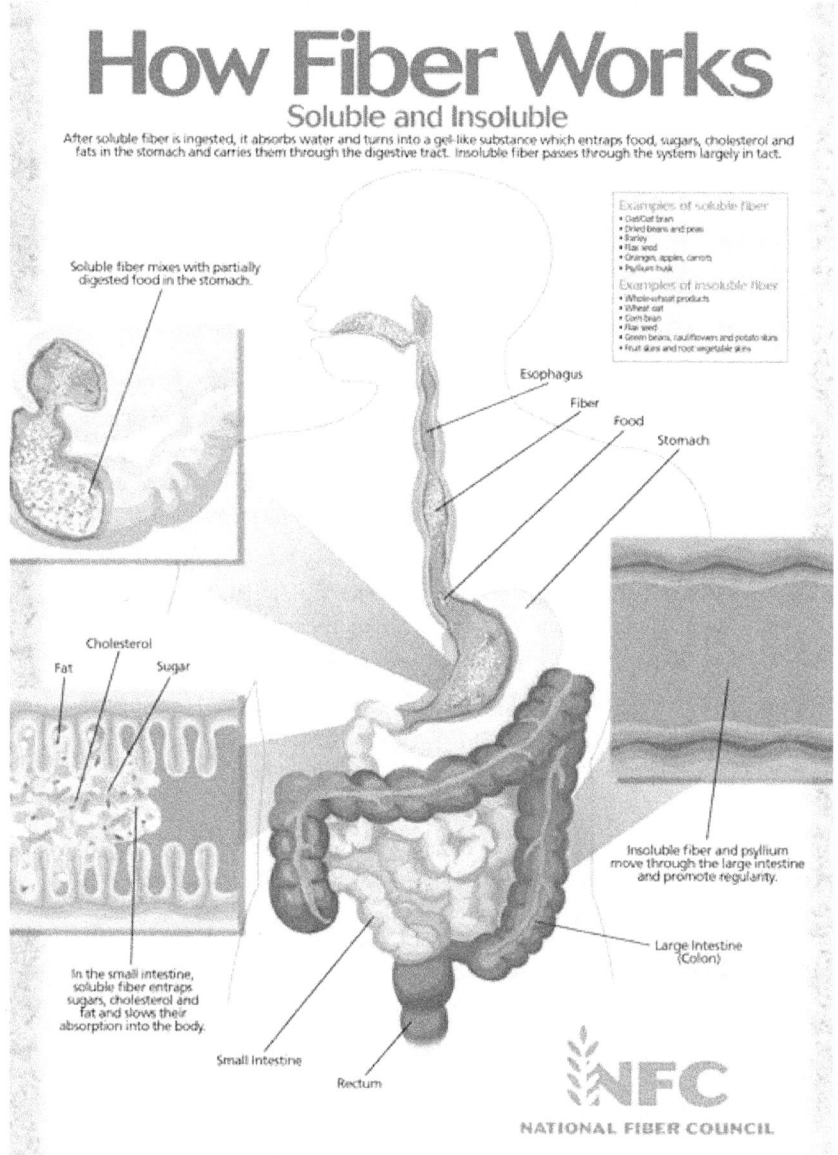

How Fiber Works
Soluble and Insoluble

After soluble fiber is ingested, it absorbs water and turns into a gel-like substance which entraps food, sugars, cholesterol and fats in the stomach and carries them through the digestive tract. Insoluble fiber passes through the system largely in tact.

Examples of soluble fiber
- Oat/Oat bran
- Dried beans and peas
- Barley
- Flax seed
- Oranges, apples, carrots
- Psyllium husk

Examples of insoluble fiber
- Whole-wheat products
- Wheat oat
- Corn bran
- Flax seed
- Green beans, cauliflower and potato skins
- Fruit skins and root vegetable skins

Soluble fiber mixes with partially digested food in the stomach.

Esophagus

Fiber

Food

Stomach

Cholesterol

Fat   Sugar

Insoluble fiber and psyllium move through the large intestine and promote regularity.

In the small intestine, soluble fiber entraps sugars, cholesterol and fat and slows their absorption into the body.

Large Intestine (Colon)

Small Intestine

Rectum

NFC
NATIONAL FIBER COUNCIL

Dietary Fiber

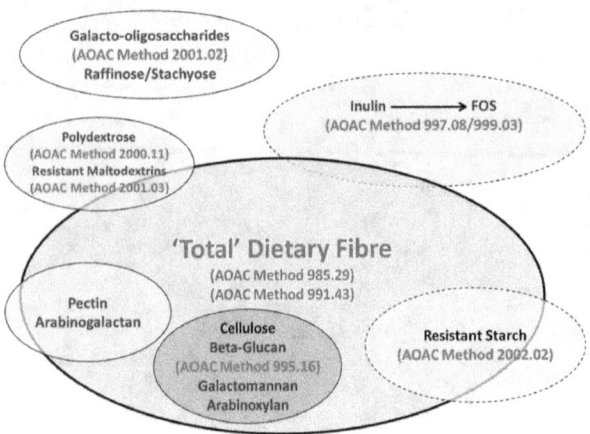

Dietary Fiber includes the non-digestible Carbohydrates and Lignin that's found intact in Plant foods. Several dietary fibers important in human nutrition are described below:

• *Cellulose:* this is the material in the Cell walls of Plants that provide structure. We find Cellulose in the Stems and Leaves of Vegetables; in the Coverings that come on Seeds and Grains, and in Skins and Hulls. Because we are unable to break down Cellulose, it remains in our Digestive Tract and contributes bulk to the food mass.

• *Hemicellulose:* This is a Polysaccharide that is also found in the Cell walls of Plants and often surrounds the Cellulose. Some Hemicelluloses help regulate our Colon pressure by providing bulk for normal Muscle action, whereas others are fermented by our Colonic Bacteria.

• *Lignin:* This is the only Dietary Fiber that is not a Carbohydrate. Ligin is a large Molecule that forms the woody part of Plants and when consumed, in our Intestine it combines with Bile Acids and prevents their reabsorption. Lignin also contributes the sandy texture found with pears and lima beans.

• *Pectin:* This is a Fiber that is also found in the Plants Cell walls. It forms a viscous, sticky gel that binds Cholesterol and prevents its absorption. Pectin also helps to slow our Gastric emptying

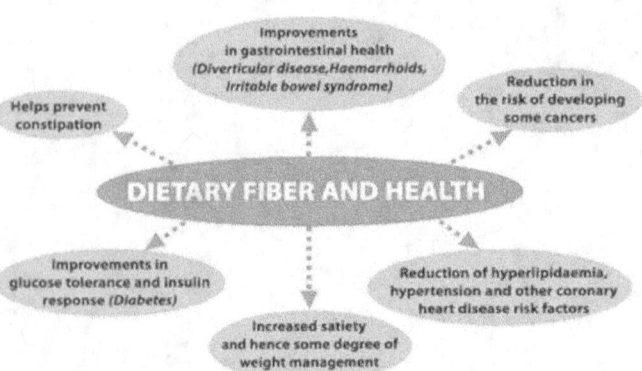

which helps to extend our feelings of satiety, allowing us to accomplish longer durations between meals. This allows our meals to be fully Digested before we eat again.

• *Gums:* When Plants are injured they respond by secreting Gums to help repair and heal itself. In our Intestine, these Gums bind Cholesterol and prevent its absorption. Bacteria in our Colon ferments these Gums to form Short-Chain Fatty Acids which help nourish our Colonic Cells.

• **β-Glucans:** These are Water-Soluble Fibers and are found in oats and oat bran, as well as manufactures food-like products that carry a health claim on the label indicating they can reduce the risk of heart disease. β-glucans interfere with the absorption of Cholesterol.

DIETARY FIBER AND ENERGY CONTENT OF SELECTED FOODS

FOOD GROUP	SERVING SIZE	DIETARY FIBER (g)	ENERGY (kcal)
Grains Group			
All Bran (wheat flakes)	¾ cup	5.0	95
Wheaties	¾ cup	2.7	95
Shredded wheat (plain)	2 biscuits	5.5	155
Instant oatmeal, cooked	1 package	4.0	150
Cheerios	1 cup	2.6	106
Air-popped popcorn	1 cup	1.2	31
Whole-wheat bread	1 slice	1.9	81
Vegetable Group			
Kidney beans, canned	½ cup	4.4	99
Green peas, frozen, cooked	½ cup	4.4	62
Corn, frozen, cooked	½ cup	2.0	66
Potato, baked, with skin	1 medium	3.8	161
Carrots, raw	1 medium	1.7	25
Broccoli, chopped, frozen, cooked	½ cup	2.8	26
Spinach, frozen, cooked	1 cup	7.0	65
Fruit Group			
Apple, with skin	1 small	3.6	77
Strawberries, sliced	1 cup	3.3	53
Orange	1 medium	3.1	62
Banana	1 medium	3.1	105

Functional Fiber

Functional Fibers are the non-digestible Polysaccharides that manufactures have added to a food-like product to increase its Fiber content.

The term *Functional Fiber* is the nutritional term used to distinguish those Fibers that are added (unnaturally) to food-like products from the naturally occurring Fibers that are intact in Plants and eaten in that form.

Functional fibers can be isolated from Plant sources/foods or manufactured, and then are used as dietary supplements or added to processed foods.

Any particular Fiber can be either a Dietary Fiber or a Functional Fiber, which depends on how it is eaten or used. The pectin in an Apple is an example of a Dietary Fiber.

In comparison, Pectin that was isolated from its natural Fruit sources and added to commercial jellies or used as a Fiber ingredient in patient tube feedings is classified as a Functional Fiber.

Functional fibers that are added in food processing must be listed on the food label. Flaxseed and Psyllium are two examples of common Functional Fibers.

Flaxseed is used as a common ingredient in breads and cereals that you find marketed as being high in Fiber. Psyllium is the main ingredient in bulk laxatives and is also available as a dietary supplement.

Foods high in Fiber are usually found to have low to moderate amounts of KCalories.

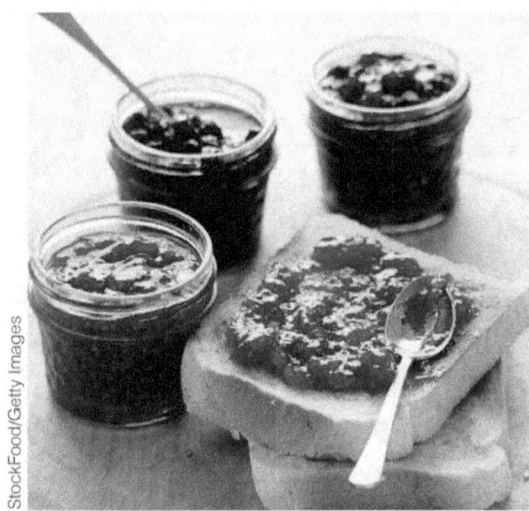

StockFood/Getty Images

a. Fiber is sometimes added to change the physical properties of foods. Pectin, which is a soluble fiber found in fruits and vegetables, is added to jams and jellies as a thickener. Gums are also used as thickeners because they combine with water to keep solutions from separating; gum arabic, gum karaya, guar gum, locust bean gum, xanthan gum, and gum tragacanth, which are extracted from shrubs, trees, and seedpods, and agar, carrageenan, and alginates, which are gums derived from seaweed, are frequently added to foods.

DIETARY FIBER AND ENERGY CONTENT OF SELECTED FOODS

FOOD GROUP	SERVING SIZE	DIETARY FIBER (g)	ENERGY (kcal)
Grains Group			
All Bran (wheat flakes)	cup	5.0	95
Wheaties	cup	2.7	95
Shredded wheat (plain)	2 biscuits	5.5	155
Instant oatmeal, cooked	1 package	4.0	150
Cheerios	1 cup	2.6	106
Air-popped popcorn	1 cup	1.2	31
Whole-wheat bread	1 slice	1.9	81
Vegetable Group			
Kidney beans, canned	cup	4.4	99
Green peas, frozen, cooked	cup	4.4	62
Corn, frozen, cooked	cup	2.0	66
Potato, baked, with skin	1 medium	3.8	161
Carrots, raw	1 medium	1.7	25
Broccoli, chopped, frozen, cooked	cup	2.8	26
Spinach, frozen, cooked	1 cup	7.0	65
Fruit Group			
Apple, with skin	1 small	3.6	77
Strawberries, sliced	1 cup	3.3	53

FOOD GROUP	SERVING SIZE	DIETARY FIBER (g)	ENERGY (kcal)
Orange	1 medium	3.1	62
Banana	1 medium	3.1	105

Data from U.S. Department of Agriculture, Agricultural Research Service. 2013. USDA National Nutrient Database for Standard Reference, Release 26. Nutrient Data Laboratory Home Page, http://www.ars.usda.gov/ba/bhnrc/ndl.

Functional Foods: Special Carbohydrate Foods

Functional foods, are described as foods that are believed to help improve our overall Health and Well-Being as well as helping us to reduce the risk of specific diseases or conditions.

Scientifically speaking, All foods are considered Functional at some Physiologic level, meaning that they provide Nutrients that furnish Energy, build or repair our Tissues, or support our Metabolic processes. But functional foods move beyond these necessary roles to provide additional health benefits.

 Although there is no regulatory definition for functional foods, this market represents about 6% of foods and beverages sold in the United States, with an annual value of $37 billion.

The first foods to be designated as Functional Foods were Carbohydrate based foods. Fruits, Vegetables, Legumes, and Grains contain tens of thousands of Phytochemicals (from the Greek word *Phyton* meaning plant).

Plants produce Phytochemicals to protect themselves against bacteria and viruses, and when the plants are eaten, these substances are absorbed and act as protective factors for humans – You ARE What You EAT!!

 Tomatoes were identified early on as a functional food because of the Lycopene they contain, which is major element in the reduction and risk of prostate cancer. Lycopene is what's known as a Carotenoid, an important Life element.

These concepts of Functional Foods or ingredients also includes new roles for familiar Nutrients. Certain Unsaturated Fatty-Acids aide in the reduction of Cardiovascular dis-ease and risk, as well as having well-known roles in maintaining our Skin integrity and providing Energy.

SELECTED FUNCTIONAL FOODS AND THEIR PROPOSED HEALTH BENEFITS

FUNCTIONAL FOOD	BIOACTIVE COMPONENT/INGREDIENT	PROPOSED HEALTH BENEFIT
Whole-grain oats	β-glucans	Reduce risk of heart disease*
Green tea	Catechins	Lower risk of certain cancers
Tomatoes	Lycopene	Lower risk of certain cancers
Fortified margarine	Plant sterols (added ingredient)	Reduce risk of heart disease*
Tree nuts	Monounsaturated fatty acids/Vitamin E	Reduce risk of heart disease*
Psyllium	Soluble fiber	Reduce risk of heart disease*

*When part of a diet low in saturated fat and cholesterol.

Adapted from American Dietetic Association: Position of the American Dietetic Association: functional foods. *J Am Diet Assoc* 109:735, 2009.

Chapter 12: Understanding Glucose

* * * * *

As we have previously discussed, the primary function of Carbohydrates is to provide us our valuable LIFE Energy, but Carbs also play other important roles in our Bodies. An example is our Nerve Tissue, they need the Sugar Galactose, and in breast-feeding women, Galactose combines with Glucose to produce the Milk Sugar Lactose.

The Monosaccharides Ribose and Deoxyribose play non-energy roles as necessary components of our RNA and DNA, respectively, the two Molecules that contain our Cell's Genetic information – our Building Blocks.

Ribose is also a component of the B Vitamin Riboflavin. Oligosaccharides are also components of our Cell Membranes, where they help signal information about our Cells, and large Polysaccharides are found in our Connective Tissue, helping provide cushioning and lubrication.

Getting Enough Glucose to Cells

Glucose is an important fuel for the Cells of our Bodies.

Many of our Cells can use Energy sources other than Glucose, but our Brain Cells, Red Blood Cells, and a few others **must** have Glucose to stay alive.

In order to provide a steady supply of Glucose, the concentration of Glucose in our Blood is regulated by our Liver and by the Hormones secreted by our Pancreas.

The rise in Blood Glucose levels after eating stimulates our Pancreas to secrete the hormone **Insulin**, which allows Glucose to enter our Muscle and Fat Cells, thereby lowering the level of Glucose in our Blood.

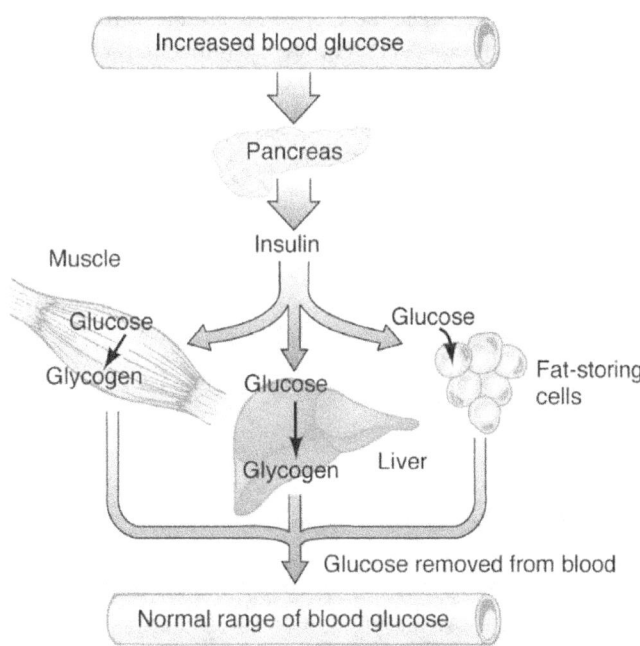

In our Muscle, Insulin stimulates the synthesis of Glycogen from the available Glucose. In our Fat-storing Cells, Insulin promotes Fat synthesis. In our Liver, Insulin promotes the storage of Glucose as Glycogen and, to a lesser extent, Fat.

Insulin also stimulates Protein synthesis. The overall effect of Insulin is to remove Glucose from our Blood and promote Energy storage.

A few hours after eating, Blood Glucose levels—and consequently the amount of Glucose that's available to our Cells—have decreased enough to cause the reaction in the Pancreas to secrete the hormone **Glucagon**.

Glucagon function to raise Blood Glucose by signaling our Liver Cells to break down this Glycogen into Glucose, which is then released into our Blood. At the same time, this Glucagon signals the Liver to synthesize new Glucose Molecules, which are also released into the Blood, causing the reaction that elevates Blood Glucose levels back to normal.

Glucagon is the Hormone produced in our Pancreas which raises Blood Glucose levels by stimulating the break-down of Liver Glycogen and the synthesis of Glucose.

Glucose as a Source of Energy

Cells use Glucose to provide Energy through the action of Cellular Respiration. This Cellular Respiration uses Oxygen to convert Glucose into Carbon Dioxide and Water while provide Energy manifested in the form of ATP.

Cellular respiration occurs inside the Cells of our body, where the reactions of Cellular Respiration split the bonds between the Carbon Atoms that form Glucose, which releases LIFE Energy that is used to synthesize ATP. These ATP is used to power the Energy-requiring processes in our bodies = **LIFE!!!**

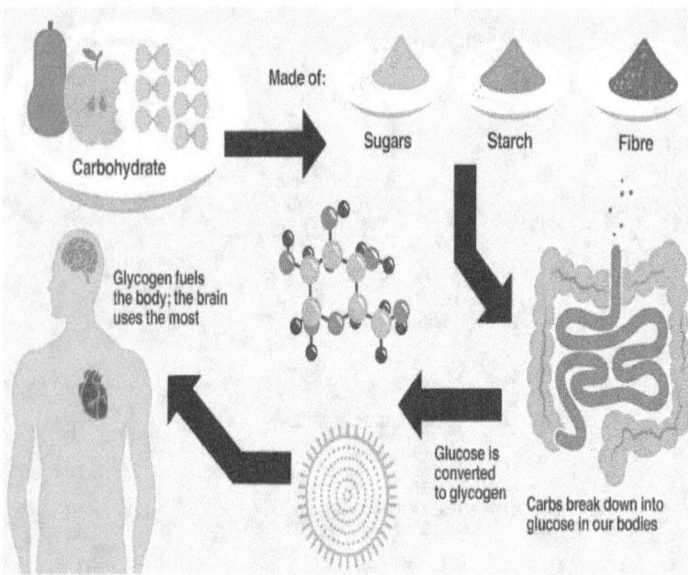

Made of:

Carbohydrate

Sugars   Starch   Fibre

Glycogen fuels the body; the brain uses the most

Glucose is converted to glycogen

Carbs break down into glucose in our bodies

The first step in our Cellular Respiration is **Glycolysis** (*glyco* = "glucose," *lysis* = "to break down").

Glycolysis can rapidly produce two Molecules of ATP from each Glucose molecule. Oxygen is not needed for this step which prompts Glycolysis to sometimes be called Anaerobic Glycolysis, or **Anaerobic Metabolism**.

When Oxygen is available, the complete breakdown of Glucose can be successfully performed.

In comparison, this **Aerobic Metabolism** produces about 36 Molecules of ATP for each Glucose molecule, 18 times more ATP than is generated by Anaerobic Glycolysis.

Glycolysis is an Anaerobic Metabolic pathway that splits Glucose into two three-Carbon Pyruvate Molecules. The energy manifested and released from one Glucose Molecule is used to make two Molecules of ATP.

Anaerobic Metabolism is metabolism with the absence of Oxygen.

Aerobic Metabolism is Metabolism in the presence of Oxygen. This is the only way our Bodies can completely break- down Glucose to manifest Carbon Dioxide, Water, and LIFE Energy in the form of ATP.

Glucose is an Essential Fuel for our Brain Cells and our Red Blood Cells.

If adequate amounts of Glucose are not available, we have an emergency feature where it can be synthesized from our Three-Carbon Pyruvate Molecules.

Carbohydrates (carbs) provide **Glucose!**

Glucose from carbs gives our body **ENERGY!**

Glucose provides:

- The **only** source of energy for the brain.

- The primary source of energy for the heart and skeletal muscles.

- When the athlete's body runs out of glucose, their muscles fatigue and performance declines QUICKLY.

**Fatty-Acids cannot be used to synthesize the Glucose we need because the reactions that break them down produce only a Two-Carbon Molecule, rather than necessary Three-Carbon one.

Some of the amino acids from Protein break-down can supply the Three-Carbon Molecules needed for Glucose synthesis.

HOWEVER, this use of our Amino Acids takes them away from our bodies needed supply of Proteins.

Our Body Proteins that are broken down to make Glucose are no longer available to perform their own job, regardless if its job is to speed up a Chemical Reaction or contract a Muscle.

A sufficient or adequate intake of dietary Carbohydrates ensures that our Protein is not utilized in this way, in this way the Carbohydrate ensures that we are successfully building and maintaining our Health and Fitness.

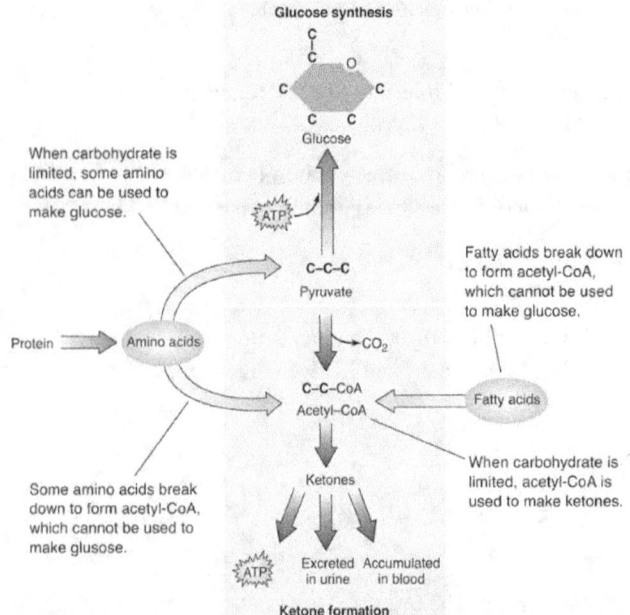

The availability of Carbohydrates in our Bodies affects the Metabolism of both Protein and Fat.

When Carbs are limited, Protein is broken down to supply Amino Acids that can be used to make Glucose.

Because the complete breakdown of Fat requires some Carbs, when Carbs are limited, Ketones are formed.

Ketones can be used as a source of Energy, but high levels can accumulate in the Blood and be excreted in the urine.

Limited or deficient intake of Carbohydrates also interferes with our Fat break-down. Most of the Energy stored in our Body is stored as Fat (Potential Energy). Fatty-Acids are broken down into Two-Carbon units that then form Acetyl-CoA.

To continue to proceed through Aerobic Metabolism, this Acetyl-CoA must combine with a Molecule that's derived primarily from a Carbohydrate. When Carbs are in a short supply, such as during starvation or when the diet is very low in carbohydrate, Acetyl-CoA Molecules cannot proceed through with the Aerobic Metabolism and instead react with each other to form the Molecules called **Ketones or Ketone Bodies.**

Our Heart, Muscles, and Kidneys can use these Ketones for Energy as an emergency or back-up.

After about three days of fasting, even our Brain has adapted and can obtain about half of its Energy from these Ketones. The use of Ketones for Energy helps spare Glucose and decreases the amount of Protein that must be broken down to synthesize Glucose.

Ketones not used for energy can be excreted in the urine. However, when Ketone production is high, they build up in the Blood, creating a condition known as **Ketosis.**

A condition of mild Ketosis can occur during starvation or especially when undertaking a low-Carb weight-loss diet and can cause symptoms that present as reduced appetite, headaches, dry mouth, and odd-smelling breath.

Severe Ketosis can occur with untreated diabetes and can increase the blood's acidity so much that normal body processes are disrupted, resulting in coma and even death.

Ketosis is a condition of having high levels of Ketones in the Blood.

Chapter 13: Carb Intake & Diabetes

* * * * *

Evidence is accumulating that show that the types of Carbohydrates consumed play a significant role in the development of Type-2 Diabetes in susceptible individuals. In populations in which the diet is high in Whole Grains, there are little to no risk of developing Type-2 Diabetes, which is the complete opposite found in populations in which the diet is high in refined starches and added sugars.

Consuming foods that are high in Refined Carbohydrates causes a greater rise in our Blood Glucose which manifests as a dangerously greater Insulin demand than consuming foods high in naturally occurring Whole Grains.

Epidemiological studies have shown that as sweetened beverage consumption increases that the risk of Diabetes has simultaneously increased along with it. Regardless of whether or not Sugar intake contributes to the development of Diabetes, diets that are high in Sugar are also high in empty KCalories, which is a significant contributor to weight gain - which __*DOES*__ increase the risk of Diabetes

Diets that are high in Un-refined Carbs from Whole Grains, Fruits, and Vegetables are always associated with a lower incidence of a variety of chronic dis-eases, whereas diets that are high in Refined Carbs, such as refined Grains and foods high in added sugars, increase chronic dis-ease

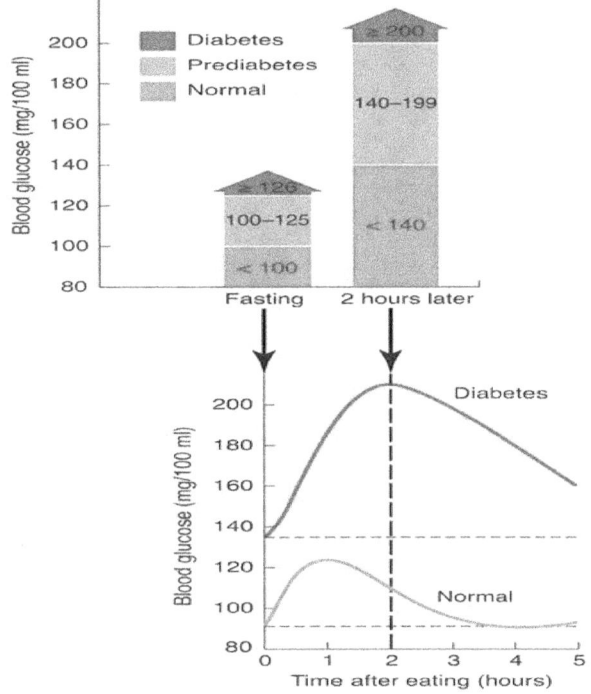

Terms such as "Low Carb" or "Net Carbs" often appear on product labels, but the Food and Drug Administration doesn't regulate these terms, so there's no standard meaning. Typically Net Carbs is used to mean the amount of Carbohydrates in a product excluding Fiber or excluding both Fiber and Sugar Alcohols.

Understanding Carbohydrates: Life Energy, Fiber, Sugar & Starch!

Most of us have heard about the Glycemic Index. The Glycemic Index classifies Carbohydrate-containing foods according to their potential to raise our Blood Sugar level.

Weight-loss diets based on the Glycemic Index typically recommend limiting foods that are higher on the Glycemic Index. Foods with a relatively high Glycemic Index ranking include potatoes and corn, and less healthy options such as 'junk' foods and desserts that contain refined flours.

Many healthy foods, such as Whole Grains, Legumes, Veggies, Fruits are naturally lower on the Glycemic Index.

Diabetes Mellitus is also commonly referred to simply as Diabetes, is classified as a dis-ease and is primarily characterized by high levels of Blood Glucose. Uncontrolled Diabetes causes damage to the Heart, Blood Vessels, Kidneys, Eyes, and Nerves and it is the leading contributing factor of adult Blindness.

Diabetes now accounts for over 44% of new cases of Kidney failure and results in more than 60% of non-traumatic lower-limb amputations. Here in the United States, over 29 million people have Diabetes, with an additional 8.1 million of these people having not been diagnosed.

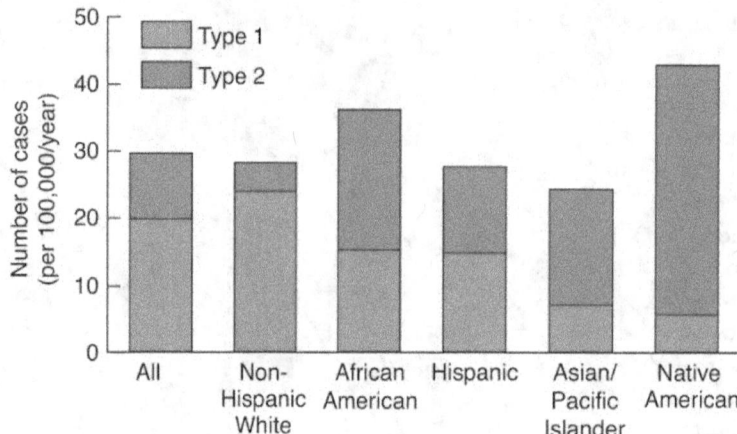

Blood Glucose levels with Diabetes

Normal Blood Glucose is less than 100 mg/100 ml Blood after an 8-hour fast; a fasting Blood level from 100 to 125 mg/100 ml is defined as prediabetes; a fasting level of 126 mg/100 ml or above is defined as Diabetes.

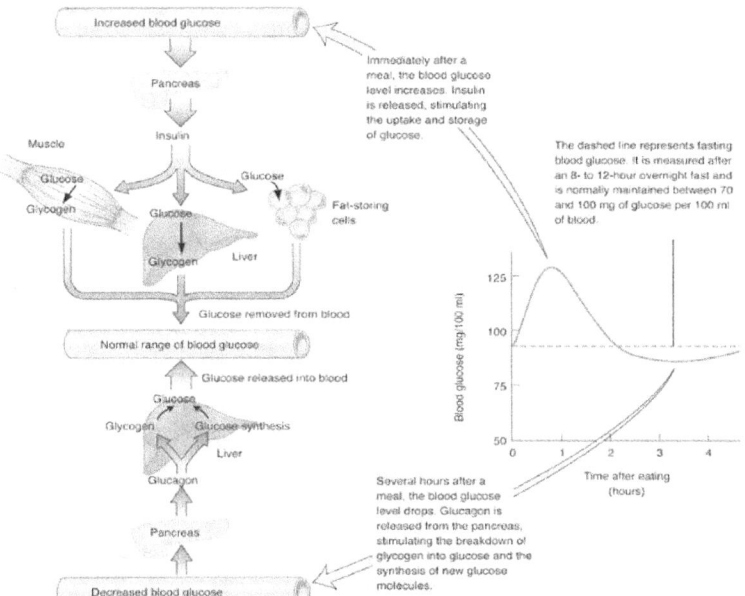

Two hours after consuming 75 g of Glucose, normal Blood levels are less than 140 mg/100 ml; prediabetes levels are from 140 to 199 mg/100 ml; Diabetes levels are 200 mg/100 ml or greater.

Types of Diabetes

Type-1 Diabetes is classified as an Autoimmune Disease in which the Insulin-secreting Pancreatic Cells are destroyed by the body's Immune System. This form of Diabetes only accounts for approximately 5 to 10% of the diagnosed cases and usually develops in someone before age 30.

Because no Insulin is produced, people with Type-1 Diabetes must inject Insulin in order to keep their Blood Glucose levels in the normal range. When their Insulin levels are low, the lack of Glucose inside the Cells leads to Ketone formation.

In uncontrolled Type-1 Diabetes, Ketone levels can get high enough to increase the Acidity of the Blood. This condition, called Diabetic Ketoacidosis and can lead to coma and death.

Type-1 Diabetes is the form of Diabetes caused by Autoimmune destruction of the Insulin-producing Cells in the Pancreas, usually leading to a state of absolute Insulin deficiency.

Autoimmune Dis-ease is a condition that results from Immune reactions that destroy normal Body Cells.

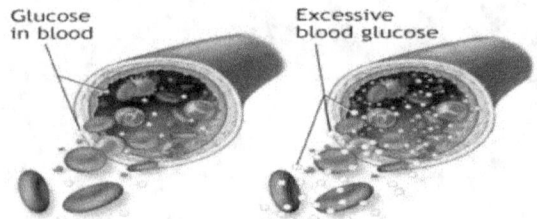

Your goal is to maintain normal blood glucose levels

Glucose in blood

Excessive blood glucose

Type-2 Diabetes is the more common form of Diabetes and this form accounts for 90 to 9.5% of all cases. It occurs when the Body does not produce enough Insulin to keep one's Blood Glucose in the normal range. This reaction can occur because Body Cells lose their sensitivity to Insulin, which is a condition called Insulin Resistance, or when the amount of Insulin that's secreted is reduced.

Type-2 diabetes is believed to be due to both genetic and lifestyle factors although its logical to focus on the lifestyle factor because it's the only one that can be effected and controlled.

Even though Type-2 Diabetes is more commonly diagnosed in adulthood, it is becoming increasingly unfortunate to find that the wrong choices are causing people can develop this Disease/condition at any age. A progressive disease, Type-2 usually begins with Pre-Diabetes, which is a condition in which Glucose levels are above normal but not high enough to be diagnosed as Diabetes. In almost ALL cases, simple adjustments in diet – switching from processed food like items to natural foods and more active lifestyle can keep Pre-Diabetes from progressing to Type-2 diabetes.

** DIABETES IS THE DIRECT RESULT OF IMPROPER EATING HABITS THAT EVENTUALLY MANIFESTS AS A DIS-EASE!

** INSTEAD OF DIABETES BEING A GENETIC PREDISPOSITION, FAMILIES SIMPLY PASS ON THE SAME EATING HABITS AND FOODS THAT CAUSE DIABETES!

** DIABETES IS A CONDITION, CALLING IT A DISEASE IS AN ILLUSION!

** REFINED SUGAR AND STARCH IN PROCESSED FOODS ARE THE DIRECT CAUSE OF DIABETES!

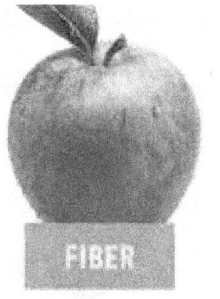

Berries

Apple

Celery

Wasa crispbreads

Wheat bran

Broccoli

Carrots

Peppers

Avocado

Chapter 14: Health Benefits of Fiber

* * * * *

Dietary Fiber directly impacts and influences the food mix in our Gastrointestinal Tract as well as the overall Gastrointestinal function. Individuals who follow dietary patterns that include higher amounts of Dietary Fiber are less likely to develop chronic conditions such as Type-2 Diabetes, cardiovascular disease, or metabolic syndrome, and they have lower mortality rates. Below is a brief outline of some of the major benefits of naturally occurring Fiber:

• *Increases fecal mass and promotes laxation:* The capacity of dietary Fiber to hold Water and Bacteria creates its bulk-forming and laxative effects. The added mass helps the food Bolus move more rapidly through our Small Intestine, promoting normal bowel action and preventing or alleviating constipation. A larger food mass in the Colon averts the development of Diverticula, small pouches that protrude outward through the lining of the Colon. When the food residue entering the Colon is low in bulk, the Muscles must then contract more forcefully to move it forward, which over time contributes to the formation of these Diverticula with risk of inflammation and infection. Dietary Fiber has been effective in treating diarrhea and may be useful in treating other Gastrointestinal conditions.

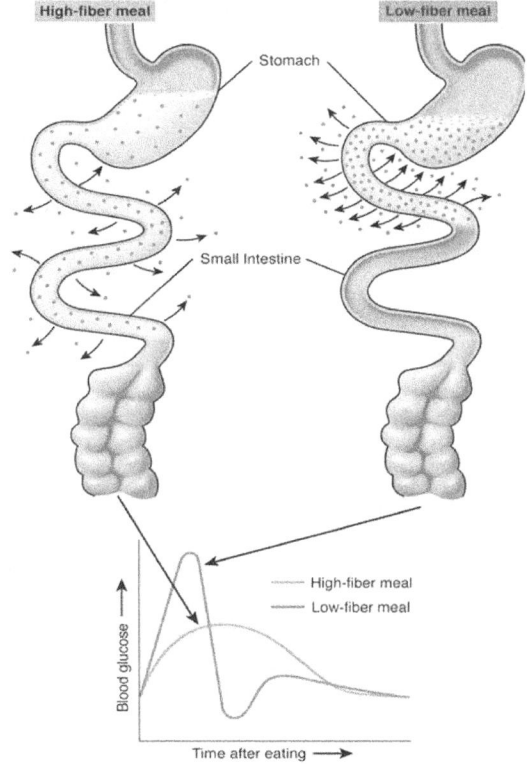

• *Promotes growth of beneficial Colonic Microflora:* Bacteria living in the Colon ferment dietary Fiber along with Resistant Starch. This action produces Short-Chain Fatty-Acids that nourish lining of our Cells of our Colon and stimulate their growth. Fiber encourages the proliferation of health-promoting Bacteria in our Colon and has been used to treat Irritable-Bowel syndrome.

• *Binds Bile Acids and Cholesterol:* Fiber binds Cholesterol and Bile Acids in the lower section of the Small Intestine and prevents their absorption. Once bound to this Fiber, Cholesterol and Bile Acids are eliminated in our feces. When Bile Acids are lost, then Cholesterol must be removed from circulating Blood Lipoproteins that would be used to synthesize their replacements, which results in a decrease in Blood Cholesterol. Ready-to-eat whole-grain oat cereal have been used to reduce LDL-Cholesterol levels.

• *Slows rise in Blood Glucose and Insulin levels:* Foods that are naturally rich in Fiber have a low GI, with their Glucose content being released slowly into the Blood. This slow release prevents a rapid spike in Blood Glucose immediately after eating. This blunting of Blood Glucose levels lessens the amount of Insulin needed to be produced to move Glucose into our Muscle and Fat Cells, which causes the reduction in the work of our Pancreas. Fiber intake at recommended levels offer major assistance in the prevention and management of Diabetes.

• *Assists in weight management:* Fiber lowers the **Energy Density** of the diet by displacing Carbohydrate, Fat, or Protein in a food, thereby causing a reduction in its Energy content. A diet containing recommended levels of Fiber also requires more mastication/chewing and in-turn promotes satiety while helping to lower food intake. The 2010 Dietary Guidelines Advisory Committee quoted strong and consistent evidence that in adults, diets lower in Energy density support weight loss and weight maintenance.

Diets lower in Energy density include more Fruits, Veggies, Whole Grains, and Legumes, and fewer KCalories from Fat, baked desserts, and fried foods. Water also lowers the Energy density of meals and particular foods, such as soups. In a national survey, individuals who consumed more Fiber in the form of Beans had lower body weights and lower waist circumferences.

Although dietary Fiber performs many actions that support our health, much remains to be learned as to its effect on specific chronic conditions. Total Fiber intake does not seem to defend against Colorectal cancer, although greater use of whole-grain cereals is associated with a lower risk of it.

It may be that other dietary components associated with Fiber—particular Nutrients or Phytochemicals—rather than the Fiber itself confer resistance to chronic dis-ease.

Heart Disease

The effect of Carbohydrate intake on Heart dis-ease and risk depends on the type of Carbs we consume. There is plenty of evidence that shoes that diets high in Sugar can and will raise Blood Lipid levels which is root cause of the increase the risk of heart disease, this is in comparison with dietary patterns that are high in Fiber from Whole Grains, Vegetables, and Fruits sharply reduce the risk of Heart disease.

We are real and naturally occurring Life forms. We NEED real and naturally occurring Foods to Replenish, Restore, Maintain and Heal ourselves – just as we are designed to do.

Dietary patterns that are high in naturally occurring Fiber is directly related to a lower rate of Heart dis-ease or risk. This is accomplished because the Fiber helps to lower Blood Cholesterol, reduce Blood Pressure, normalize Blood Glucose levels, and prevent obesity, as well as by affecting a number of other parameters that impact Heart dis-ease risk.

Soluble Fiber from foods such as Legumes, Oats, Flaxseed, and Brown Rice aide in the ability to lower and maintain Blood Cholesterol levels in a variety of beneficial ways. In our Digestive Tract, this Soluble Fiber helps eliminate Cholesterol from our Body by binding this dietary Cholesterol with our Bile Acids (which are made from Cholesterol) and this prevents the dietary Cholesterol from being absorbed. Soluble Fiber also helps lower Blood Cholesterol because it lowers Insulin levels and is broken down by Bacteria in our Colon. The resultant lower Insulin levels and the by-products of the Bacterial breakdown contribute to the inhibition of Cholesterol synthesis in our Liver.

Insoluble Fibers, such as Wheat Bran and Cellulose, are also integral and beneficial for our Heart health, but they have less of an effect on Blood Cholesterol.

** In the absence of Soluble Fiber, dietary Cholesterol and Bile, which also contains Cholesterol and Bile Acids made from Cholesterol, are able to be absorbed into the Blood and transported to the Liver for dispersal and use in the Body.

** When Soluble Fiber is present in the Digestive Tract, the Fiber binds to the dietary Cholesterol and the Bile Acids so that they are able to be excreted rather than absorbed. This is how we naturally and successfully reduce and maintain the amount of Cholesterol in the Body.

Soluble Fiber helps lower Blood Cholesterol by increasing excretion of both Bile Acids and Cholesterol.

Bowel Health

Fiber and other indigestible Carbohydrates add bulk and absorb water in our Gastrointestinal

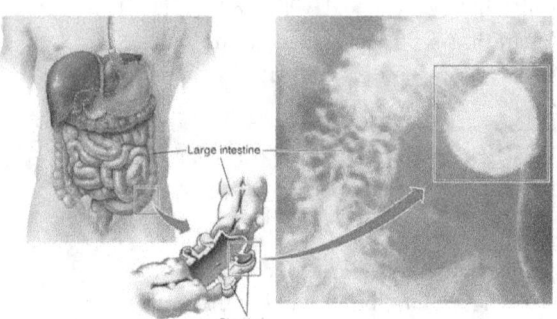

Tract, which makes our feces larger and softer while reducing the pressure needed for defecation. This helps reduce the incidence of Constipation and/or Hemorrhoids - the swelling of the Veins in the Rectal or Anal area. It also reduces the risk of developing out-pouches in the wall of the Colon called Diverticula (singular term is *Diverticulum*).

Fecal matter that has a chance to collect and sit in the GI Tract can accumulate in these pouches, causing irritation, pain, and inflammation—a condition known as Diverticulitis.

Diverticulitis may lead to an infection that presents as Inflammation in the Intestine. The treatment of it usually includes antibiotics to eliminate the infection and a limited duration of a low-Fiber diet to prevent any irritation of the inflamed tissues.

Once the inflammation is resolved, a return to high-Fiber diet is recommended to ease stool elimination and reduce future attacks of Diverticulitis.

Diverticulosis is a condition in which out-pouches form in the wall of the Colon. These Diverticula manifest at weak points of the tissue due to pressure exerted when the Colon contracts.

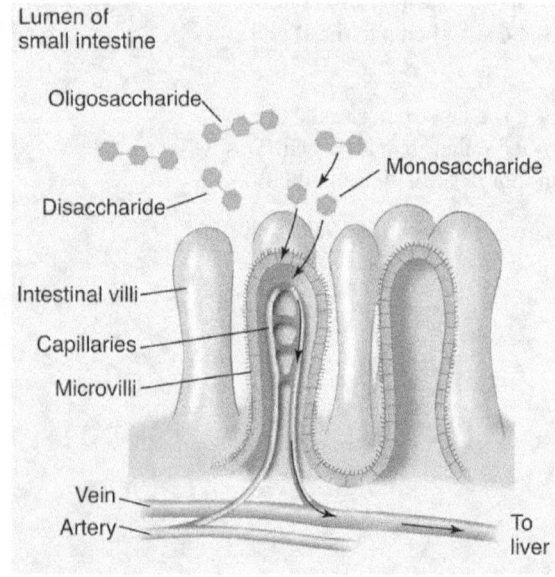

Although Fiber does speed the movement of the Intestinal contents, when the diet is low in fluid, Fiber can contribute to Constipation.

Consequently, the more Fiber in the diet equates to more water that is needed to keep the stool soft. When too little fluid is consumed, the stool becomes hard and difficult to eliminate.

In severe cases of excessive Fiber intake and low fluid intake, Intestinal blockage can occur.

A diet high in Fiber, particularly from naturally occurring whole grains, may reduce the risk of colon cancer, although not all studies support this finding.

Fiber reduces contact between the Cells lining the Colon and potentially cancer-causing substances in the feces. Fiber in the Colon also affects the Intestinal Microflora and their by-products. These by-products may directly affect Colon Cells or may change the environment of the Colon in a way that can affect the development of Colon cancer.

Some of the protective effect may also be due to Antioxidant Vitamins and Phytochemicals present in Fiber-rich whole grains.

The National Academy of Sciences' Institute of Medicine gives the following daily total fiber recommendations for adults:

	Age 50 and younger	Age 51 and older
Men	38 grams	30 grams
Women	25 grams	21 grams

Foods with Soluble and Insoluble Fiber

Soluble Fiber	Insoluble Fiber
• Apples	• Whole grain
• Pears	• Whole wheat breads
• Oranges	• Barley
• Peaches	• Brown rice
• Grapes	• Bulgur
• Prunes	• Whole-grain breakfast cereals
• Blueberries	• Wheat bran
• Strawberries	• Seeds
• Seeds and Nuts	• Vegetables:
• Oat bran	— Carrots
• Dried beans	— Cucumbers
• Oatmeal	— Zucchini
• Barley	— Celery
• Rye	— Tomatoes
• Vegetables	

Foods with High Fiber

Vegetables	Serving Size	Total fiber (grams)
Peas	1 cup	8.8
Potato, baked with skin	1 medium	4.4
Corn	1 cup	4.2
Popcorn, air-popped	3 cups	3.6
Tomato paste	¼ cup	3.0
Carrot	1 medium	2.0
Fruits	**Serving Size**	**Total fiber (grams)**
Apple, with skin	1 medium	4.4
Apricots, dried	10 halves	2.6
Raisins	1.5 ounce box	1.6
Orange	1 medium	3.1
Peaches, dried	3 halves	3.2
Blueberries	1 cup	3.5
Pear	1 medium	5.1
Legumes, Nuts & Seeds	**Serving Size**	**Total Fiber (grams)**
Cashews	18 nuts	0.9
Peanuts	28 nuts	2.3
Pistachio nuts	47 nuts	2.9
Almonds	24 nuts	3.3
Baked beans, canned	1 cup	10.4
Lima beans	1 cup	13.2
Black beans	1 cup	15.0
Lentils	1 cup	15.6
Grains, Cereal & Pasta	**Serving Size**	**Total Fiber (grams)**
Bread, mixed grain	1 slice	1.7
Bread, whole-wheat	1 slice	1.9
Bread, rye	1 slice	1.9
Oatmeal	1 cup	4.0
Bran flakes	¾ cup	5.1
Spaghetti, whole-wheat	1 cup	6.3

Chapter 15: Non-Nutritive Sweeteners

* * * * *

The FDA has approved Saccharin, Aspartame, Sucralose, Acesulfame K, Neotame, and Stevia as Non-nutritive Sweeteners and defined the Acceptable Daily Intakes (ADIs)—levels that can be consumed daily over a lifetime without appreciable health risk (Table).

Nonnutritive Sweeteners

Sweetener	Brand names	What is it?	ADI
Saccharin	Sweet'N Low, SugarTwin	The oldest of the nonnutritive sweeteners, developed in 1879. It was once considered a carcinogen but was taken off the government's list of cancer-causing substances in 2000. It is 300 times sweeter than sucrose and has a bitter aftertaste.	5 mg/kg of body weight/day; one packet contains 20 mg of saccharin. Beverages are limited to < 12 mg/fluid ounce. A 154-lb (70-kg) person would exceed the ADI by consuming 18 packets.
Aspartame	Equal, NutraSweet	Made of two amino acids (phenylalanine and aspartic acid). Because it breaks down when heated, it is typically used in cold products or added after cooking. It is 200 times sweeter than sucrose.	50 mg/kg of body weight/day; one packet contains 37 mg of aspartame. To exceed the ADI, a 154-lb (70-kg) person would have to consume 95 packets or 16 12-oz aspartame-sweetened beverages. It must be limited in the diets of people with phenylketonuria.
Acesulfame K	Sunett, Sweet One	A heat-stable sweetener that is often used in combination with other sweeteners. It is 200 times sweeter than sucrose.	15 mg/kg of body weight/day; a 154-lb (70-kg) person could consume 2 gallons of beverages containing acesulfame K without exceeding the ADI.
Neotame	Neotame is not sold as a tabletop sweetener.	Made from the same two amino acids as aspartame, but because the bond between them is harder to break than the bond in aspartame, it is heat stable and can be used in baking. It is used in soft drinks, dairy products, and gum but is not sold as a tabletop sweetener. It is 8000 times sweeter than sucrose.	18 mg/kg of body weight/day.
Sucralose	Splenda	Made from sucrose molecules that have been modified so that they cannot be digested or absorbed. It is heat stable so it can be used in cooking. It is 600 times sweeter than sucrose.	5 mg/kg of body weight/day; one packet contains about 12 mg of sucralose. A 154-lb (70-kg) person could consume 29 packets without exceeding the ADI.
Stevia		A natural sweetener made from the leaf of the stevia plant.[22] It is the newest sweetener on the market and is about 250 times sweeter than sucrose.	4 mg/kg of body weight/day; to exceed the ADI, a 154-lb (70-kg) person would have to consume more than 10 packets of a stevia

Sweetener	Brand names	What is it?	ADI
	Truvia, Pure Via		sweetener or drink about six 12-oz cans of a stevia-sweetened soda.

****NON-NUTRITIVE IS A CATCH-PHRASE FOR TOXIC !!!****

When these TOXIC non-nutritive sweeteners are used to replace added Sugars in the diet, they significantly increase the incidences of Dental Caries and severely hamper the ability to manage Blood Sugar levels.

Whether the use of these products promotes weight loss, however, depends on whether the KCalories they spare are added back from other food sources. Studies on the effects of these TOXIC non-nutritive sweeteners on body weight have had mixed results.

Animal studies suggest that these TOXIC artificial sweeteners may stimulate appetite, leading to weight gain, but this hypothesis has not been supported by studies done in humans. Weight gain seen in some studies of artificial sweetener users is more likely to be due to the fact that individuals at higher risk of obesity are more likely to use artificial sweeteners to try to control weight.

If you think switching to nonnutritive sweeteners will make your diet healthier, think again. Foods that are high in added sugar tend to be Nutrient DEFICIENT. Replacing them with artificially sweetened alternatives does not necessarily increase the Nutrient density of the diet or improve overall diet quality.

IN FACT, THESE ITEMS INCREASE THE LEVEL OF TOXICITY IN THE DIET!

High-fructose corn syrup (HFCS) is the most common added sweetener in the American diet. The ubiquitous use of this sweetener has created concern about the effect it has on our health. Increased consumption of HFCS has been implicated in the development of obesity, heart disease, and diabetes, among other disorders.

Is HFCS just a convenient way to sweeten our food, or is it a threat to our health?

HFCS is a syrup made by extracting starch from corn and treating it to break the Bonds between the Glucose Molecules. The resulting Corn Syrup is then treated to convert about half the Glucose to Fructose (hence "high-fructose" corn syrup).

Manufacturers prefer HFCS as an added sweetener because it is cheaper and more stable during storage than other sweeteners. In 1970, the most common sweetener in the American diet was Sucrose (see graph below). Today HFCS has almost completely replaced sucrose in soft drinks and is found in many other foods, ranging from breakfast cereals to canned soups and salad dressings.

HFCS has been implicated in the growing obesity crisis because the increase in its use parallels the increase in obesity (see graph).

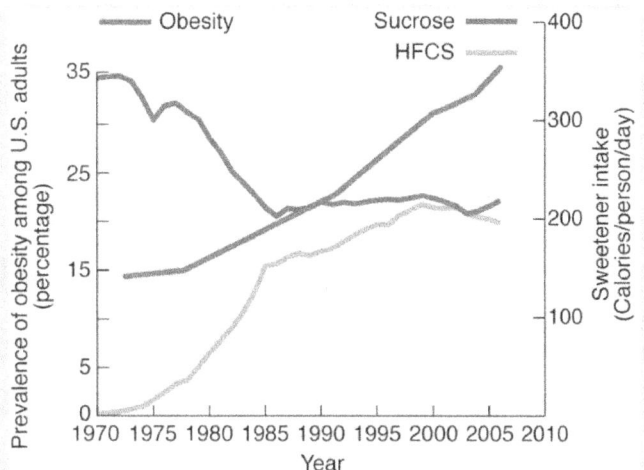

Obesity in turn increases the risk of diabetes and Heart disease. There is a physiological basis for a relationship between Fructose and obesity. When excess energy is consumed, Fructose is converted to Fat more readily than Glucose.

Since 1970, HFCS intake has increased dramatically, while sucrose use has declined. Over this same time period, the incidence of obesity has more than doubled.

In addition, Fructose is not as effective as Glucose at stimulating the release of Hormones that suppress appetite or at inhibiting the release of Hormones that stimulate appetite. So, when compared to Glucose, Fructose consumption contributes more to Fat synthesis and less to appetite suppression, potentially leading to overeating and weight gain.

A study in humans found a greater amount of abdominal fat in subjects consuming diets high in Fructose compared to Glucose.

There are a number of counterarguments to the contention that HFCS contributes to obesity more than other sweeteners. First, obesity has increased dramatically in countries that do not use HFCS, and in the United States obesity rates continued to increase even after HFCS consumption leveled off.

The most compelling argument as to why HFCS is not to blame for obesity is that it is really no different than Sucrose. Sucrose is 50% Fructose, while the HFCS used in soft drinks is about 55% Fructose. There is no Metabolic reason why the fructose in HFCS is more damaging than the Fructose in Sucrose, unless the slight difference in the amount of Fructose in these two sweeteners is metabolically significant.

In an animal study, rats fed a diet supplemented with water sweetened with HFCS gained more weight and more Fat than the rats supplemented with Sucrose-sweetened water, despite actually consuming fewer calories.

However, studies in Humans have found responses to consumption of HFCS and Sucrose to be the same with regard to its biologic actions and effect on food intake. In a study of weight-loss diets containing 20% of KCalories from HFCS or Sucrose, similar weight changes were seen.

Is HFCS worse than other sweeteners? We gain excess body weight by consuming more energy than we expend. Calories from beverages, whether sweetened with sucrose or HFCS, are a particular concern because the added calories are not compensated for by reductions in solid food intake. Numerous studies have shown a positive association between sweetened beverage consumption and the risk of obesity in adults.

When consumed in large amounts, HFCS has the potential to both increase energy intake and promote the deposition of body fat. But will eliminating HFCS from our food supply necessarily make our diets healthier? Will replacing HFCS with sucrose help reduce obesity?

A large range of processed foods, from carbonated beverages and fruit drinks to cereals, crackers, barbeque sauce, and salad dressings, contain high-fructose corn syrup.

Since 1970, the intake of HFCS has increased dramatically, while Sucrose use has declined. Over this same time period the incidence of Obesity has more than doubled.

PROPERTIES AND APPLICATIONS OF COMMON NONNUTRITIVE SWEETENERS

NAME	SWEETENING POWER (COMPARED WITH SUCROSE)	EFFECT OF HEAT	TRADE NAMES	APPLICATIONS
Aspartame	160-220 times sweeter	Degrades during heating and loses sweetening power	NutraSweet, Equal, Sugar Twin (blue box)	Beverages, table sweetener, gelatin, pudding, chewing gum, cold breakfast cereal
Acesulfame-K	200 times sweeter	Stable at baking temperatures	Sweet One, Sweet & Safe	Beverages, table sweetener, baked goods, all-purpose sweetener; excluded for use in meat and poultry
Saccharin"	300 times sweeter	Not affected by heat	Sweet and Low, Sweet Twin, Necta Sweet, Sweet 'N Low Brown	Beverages, table sweetener, chewing gum, baked goods, pudding
Sucralose	600 times sweeter	Not affected by heat in cooking and baking	Splenda	Beverages, desserts, baked goods, candy, table sweetener, all-purpose sweetener
Neotame	7000-13,000 times sweeter	Not affected by heat	Little used in food processing	Approved for general use except for meat and poultry
Stevia (steviol glycosides-rebaudioside A extracted from stevia plant leaves)	250 times sweeter	Shelf-stable in dry forms or liquids	Truvia, Rebiana, PureVia, SweetLeaf	Beverages, cereals, energy bars, table sweetener
Luo Han Guo extract	150-300 times sweeter	May have an aftertaste at high levels	Not commonly used	Table top sweetener, general food ingredient, use with other sweetener blends

Summary

* * * * *

We have the potential to Live until we literally don't want to live anymore. As the explore and discovery Ancient Civilizations, they are finding Bones that carbon-date into the MILLIONS of years old. This is an in-sight into the considerable Life-Span that we can actively achieve !

Life is Energy. Our #1 Food-Energy Source is manifested in the Molecular form of Carbohydrates. So , when we focus on Nutrition and dietary choices, our #1 Energy source should be our Primary Focus.

The first step in achieving our physical potential and Greatness is n Understanding our FOOD. We can only do one of two things – eat to die or EAT TO LIVE !

We are Created with the BEST vehicle in the Universe....which is PERFECT......and all we have to do is operate according and we gain the ability to Manifest and Express the Highest Quality of Humanity = The Image & Likeness of THE CREATOR !!!!

CARBOHYDRATES ARE SUNLIGHT IN ATOMIC FORM !!!!!!!!!!!!!!!!

CARBOHYDRATES IS HOW WE EAT THE SUN !!!!!!!!!!!!!!!!!!!

OUR CELLS NEED 2 ELEMENTS FOR GROWTH & DEVELOPMENT = OXYGEN & GLUCOSE (CARBOHYDRATES) !!!!!!!!!!!!!!!!!!

Abundant LIFE is within our grasp and is ours to EASILY achieve and maintain = IT'S OUR DESTINY !!!!!!

Life is ENERGY

The SUN is our Source of Life Energy

We ARE what we EAT

The Plants use the process of Photosynthesis to Transform the un-seen Life Energy of the SUN into the Atomic composition of CARBOHYDRATES, so that when we Digest the Plants, our Bodies release the Life/Sun Energy to LIVE !!!!!

1. **Carbohydrates in Our Food**

   o   Unrefined Whole Grains, Fruits, and Vegetables are good sources of our Fiber and
   Micronutrients. When these foods are refined, these valuable Nutrients and Fiber
   are destroyed/lost. Whole grains contain the entire Kernel, which includes the
   Endosperm, Bran, and Germ. Refined grains include only the Endosperm. Refined
   grains are enriched with some of the B vitamins and Iron, but not all the nutrients
   lost in refining are added back.

   Whole grains

   o   Refined sugars contain calories but few Nutrients; for this reason, foods high in
   added refined sugar are low in Nutrient density.

2. **Types of Carbohydrates**

   o   Carbohydrates contain Carbon as well as h\Hydrogen and Oxygen, in the same
   proportion as Water. Simple Carbohydrates include Monosaccharides and
   Disaccharides and are found in foods such as table sugar, honey, milk, and fruit.
   Complex Carbohydrates are Polysaccharides; they include Glycogen in animals and
   Starches and the Fiber in plants.

   Carbohydrate structures and sources

   o   Fiber cannot be digested in the stomach or small intestine and therefore is not
   absorbed into the body. Soluble fiber dissolves in water to form a viscous solution
   and is digested by bacteria in the colon; insoluble fiber is not readily digested by
   bacteria and adds bulk to fecal matter.

3. **Carbohydrate Digestion and Absorption**

   o   Disaccharides and Starches must be digested to Monosaccharides before they can
   be absorbed. In individuals with Lactose intolerance, Lactose passes into the Colon
   undigested, causing cramps, gas, and diarrhea. Indigestible Complex
   Carbohydrates, including Fiber, some Oligosaccharides, and Resistant Starch, can
   increase intestinal gas, but they benefit health by increasing bulk in the stool,
   promoting growth of healthy Microflora, and slowing nutrient absorption.

   Carbohydrate digestion

   o   After a meal, Blood Glucose levels rise. The rate, magnitude, and duration of this
   rise are referred to as the Glycemic Response. Glycemic Response is affected by
   the amount and type of Carbohydrate consumed and by other nutrients ingested
   with the carbohydrate.

4. Carbohydrate Functions

- o Carbohydrate, primarily as Glucose, provides Energy to the body. Blood Glucose levels are maintained by the Hormones Insulin and Glucagon. When Blood Glucose levels rise Insulin from the Pancreas allows Muscle and fat-storing cells to take up Glucose from the Blood and promotes the synthesis of Glycogen, Fat, and Protein. When Blood Glucose levels fall, Glucagon increases them by causing Glycogen breakdown and Glucose synthesis.

Blood glucose regulation

- o Glucose is metabolized through Cellular Respiration. It begins with Glycolysis, which breaks each six-Carbon Glucose molecule into two three-Carbon Pyruvate Molecules, producing ATP even when Oxygen is unavailable. The complete breakdown of Glucose through Aerobic Metabolism requires Oxygen and produces Carbon Dioxide, Water, and more ATP than Glycolysis.

- o When Carbohydrate intake is limited, Amino Acids from the breakdown of body Proteins can be used to synthesize Glucose. Therefore, an adequate Carbohydrate intake is said to spare Protein. Limited Carbohydrate intake also results in the formation of Ketones (Ketone Bodies) by the Liver. These can be used as an Energy source by other Tissues. Ketones that accumulate in the Blood can cause symptoms that range from headache and lack of appetite to coma and even death if levels are extremely high.

5. Carbohydrates in Health and Disease

- o **Diabetes mellitus** is characterized by high Blood Glucose levels, that occur either because insufficient Insulin is produced or because of a decrease in the body's sensitivity to Insulin. Over time, high Blood Glucose levels damage tissues and contribute to the development of heart disease, kidney failure, blindness, and infections that may lead to amputations. Treatment includes diet, exercise, and medication to keep Glucose levels in the normal range.

Blood glucose levels in diabetes

- o **Hypoglycemia**, or low Blood Glucose, causes symptoms such as sweating, headaches, and rapid heartbeat.

- o Diets high in Carbohydrate, particularly Sucrose, increase the risk of Dental Caries. Sucrose helps bacteria to stick to the Teeth, and they then use Sucrose and other Carbohydrates as a food supply, producing Acids that damage the Teeth.

- o Gram for gram, Carbohydrates provide less Energy than Fat. High-Fiber diets can prevent weight gain by making you feel full longer so that you eat less. Low-Carbohydrate diets promote weight loss by causing a spontaneous reduction in food intake. Non-nutritive sweeteners aid weight loss if the Sugar calories they replace are not added back from other food sources.

o   Diets high in unrefined Carbohydrates from whole grains, vegetables, fruits, and legumes may reduce the risk of heart disease, bowel disorders, and colon cancer. Soluble Fiber helps prevent heart disease because it can lower Blood Cholesterol.

6. **Meeting Carbohydrate Needs**

o   Guidelines for a healthy diet recommend 45 to 65% of Energy from Carbohydrates. Most of this should come from whole grains, legumes, fruits, and vegetables. Foods high in added sugar should

be consumed in moderation.

Facts and Figures

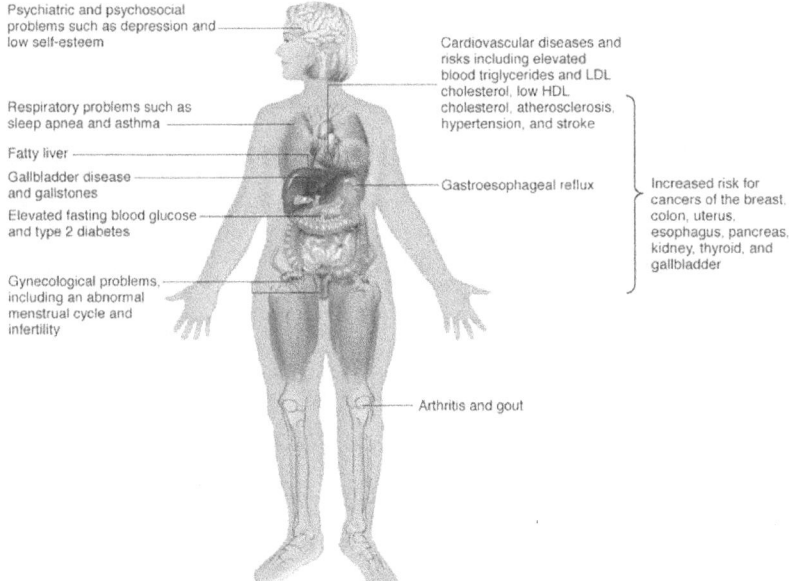

Psychiatric and psychosocial problems such as depression and low self-esteem

Cardiovascular diseases and risks including elevated blood triglycerides and LDL cholesterol, low HDL cholesterol, atherosclerosis, hypertension, and stroke

Respiratory problems such as sleep apnea and asthma

Fatty liver

Gallbladder disease and gallstones

Gastroesophageal reflux

Increased risk for cancers of the breast, colon, uterus, esophagus, pancreas, kidney, thyroid, and gallbladder

Elevated fasting blood glucose and type 2 diabetes

Gynecological problems, including an abnormal menstrual cycle and infertility

Arthritis and gout

Health consequences of Excess Body Fat (Potential Energy)

Obesity-related health complications such as those highlighted here have reached epidemic proportions in the United States and around the world.

Being overweight also has psychological and social consequences. Overweight and obese individuals of any age are at increased risk of experiencing depression, negative self-image, and feelings of inadequacy.

They may also be discriminated against in college admissions, in the workplace, and even on public transportation. The physical health consequences of excess body Fat may not manifest themselves as disease for years, but the psychological and social problems are experienced every day.

Because obesity increases health problems, it increases health care costs. Estimates suggest that obesity "costs" about $147 billion per year.[4]The greater the number of obese people, the higher the nation's health care expenses and the higher the cost to society as a whole in terms of lost wages and productivity.

Excess Fat in the Visceral region increases health risks. Waist circumference measurements can help assess risk.

Where your extra fat is deposited is determined primarily by your genes. Age, gender, ethnicity, and lifestyle also influence where fat is stored. Visceral Fat storage increases with age.

Excess Visceral Fat is more common in men than in women, but after menopause, the amount of Visceral Fat in women increases.

Caucasians and Asians have more Visceral Fat than African Americans with similar amounts of body Fat.

Stress, tobacco use, and alcohol consumption predispose people to Visceral Fat deposition, and weight loss and exercise reduce the amount of Visceral Fat.

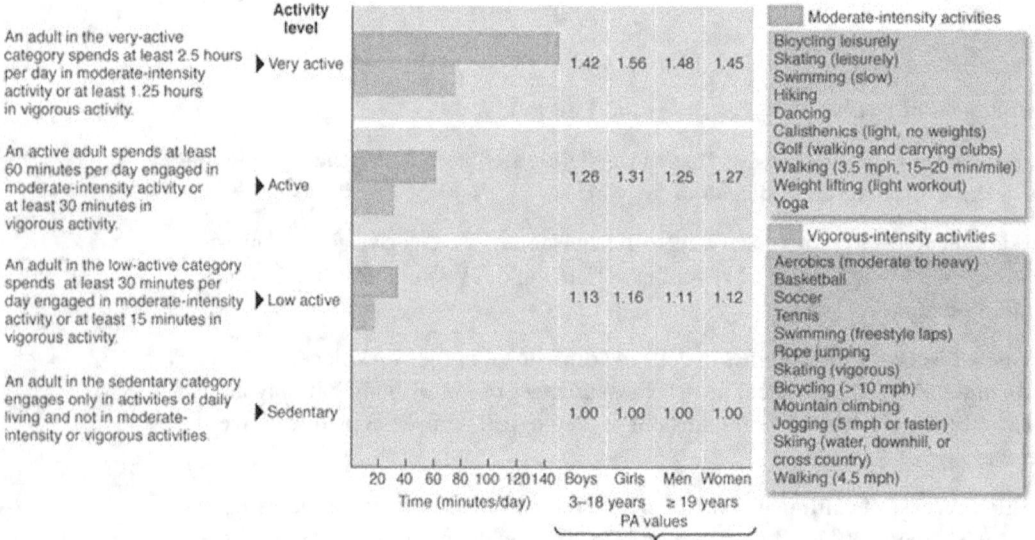

Each physical activity level is assigned a numerical physical activity (PA) value that can then be used in the EER calculation.

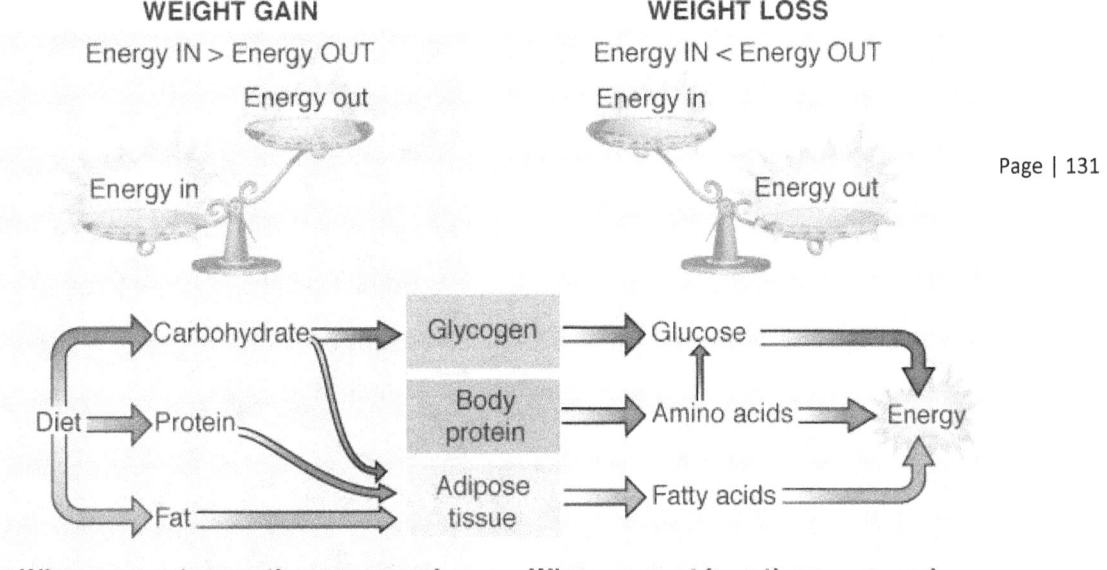

Energy balance: Storing and retrieving energy

When Calories are consumed in excess of our needs, they are transferred and stored, mostly as Fat (Potential Energy). If the excess Calories are consumed as Fat, they are more easily transferred and stored as body Fat. If the excess Calories are consumed as Carbohydrate, they are transferred and stored as Glycogen (Potential Energy) or also converted into Fat. If excess Calories are consumed as Protein, they are converted into body Fat. When Calorie intake is less than needs, Energy can be retrieved from these stores of Potential Energy or Body Fat.

Glycogen (Potential Energy) and Body Proteins can be broken down to supply Glucose........ and Triglycerides in Adipose Tissue can be broken down to supply Fatty Acids.

Stored Energy is used when Energy intake is reduced, both in the short term, such as when you haven't eaten a meal for a few hours, and in the long term, such as when you are trying to lose weight. To maintain a steady supply of Blood Glucose, Liver Glycogen is broken-down.

Although Protein is not considered a form of Stored Energy, when our Energy needs are not met, our Body Protein, primarily Muscle Protein, can be broken-down to yield Amino Acids, which can then be used to manifest Glucose or produce ATP. Energy for Tissues that don't require Glucose is provided by the break-down of stored Fat (triglycerides). Nutrients consumed in the next meal replenish these stores, but with prolonged Energy restriction, Fat (Potential Energy) and Protein are lost, and body weight is reduced. It is estimated that an Energy deficit of about 3500 Calories results in the loss of a pound of Adipose Tissue.

DRI recommended intake tables for Vitamins and for Minerals are on the front and back covers of this text.

Acceptable Macronutrient Distribution Ranges (AMDR) for Healthy Diets as a Percent of Energy

Source: Institute of Medicine, Food and Nutrition Board. "Dietary Reference Intakes for Energy, Carbohydrates, Fiber, Fat, Fatty Acids, Cholesterol, Protein, and Amino Acids." Washington, D.C.: National Academies Press, 2002, 2005.

Age	Carbohydrate	Added Sugars	Total Fat	Linoleic Acid	α-Linolenic Acid	Protein
1–3 y	45–65	≤25	30–40	5–10	0.6–1.2	5–20
4–18 y	45–65	≤25	25–35	5–10	0.6–1.2	10–30
≥19 y	45–65	≤25	20–35	5–10	0.6–1.2	10–35

Dietary Reference Intakes: Recommended Intakes for Individuals: Carbohydrates, Fiber, Fat, Fatty Acids, Protein, and Water

Source: Institute of Medicine, Food and Nutrition Board. "Dietary Reference Intakes for Energy, Carbohydrate, Fiber, Fat, Fatty Acids, Cholesterol, Protein, and Amino Acids" (2002/2005); "Dietary Reference Intakes for Water, Potassium, Sodium, Chloride, and Sulfate" (2005) Washington, D.C.: National Academies Press.

Life Stage Group	Carbohydrate (g/day)	Fiber (g/day)	Fat (g/day)	Linoleic Acid (g/day)	α-Linolenic Acid (g/day)	Protein (g/kg/day)[a]	(g/day)	Water[b] (L/day)
Infants								
0–6 mo	60*	ND	31*	4.4*†	0.5*‡	1.52*	9.1*	0.7*
6–12 mo	95*	ND	30*	4.6*†	0.5*‡	1.50	11.0	0.8*
Children								
1–3 y	130	19*	ND	7*	0.7*	1.10	13	1.3*
4–8 y	130	25*	ND	10*	0.9*	0.95	19	1.7*
Males								
9–13 y	130	31*	ND	12*	1.2*	0.95	34	2.4*
14–18 y	130	38*	ND	16*	1.6*	0.85	52	3.3*
19–30 y	130	38*	ND	17*	1.6*	0.80	56	3.7*
31–50 y	130	38*	ND	17*	1.6*	0.80	56	3.7*
51–70 y	130	30*	ND	14*	1.6*	0.80	56	3.7*
>70 y	130	30*	ND	14*	1.6*	0.80	56	3.7*
Females								
9–13 y	130	26*	ND	10*	1.0*	0.95	34	
14–18y	130	26*	ND	11*	1.1*	0.85	46	2.1*
19–30 y	130	25*	ND	12*	1.1*	0.80	46	2.3*
31–50 y	130	25*	ND	12*	1.1*	0.80	46	2.7*
51–70 y	130	21*	ND	11*	1.1*	0.80	46	2.7*
>70 y	130	21*	ND	11*	1.1*	0.80	46	2.7*
Pregnancy	175	28*	ND	13*	1.4*	1.10	71	3.0*
Lactation	210	29*	ND	13*	1.3*	1.10	71	3.8*

ND = not determined.

*Values are AI (Adequate Intakes).

†Refers to all ω-6 polyunsaturated fatty acids.

‡Refers to all ω-3 polyunsaturated fatty acids.

[a] Based on g protein per kg of body weight for the reference body weight, e.g., for adults 0.8 g/kg body weight for the reference body weight.

[b] Total water includes all water contained in food, beverages, and drinking water.

EXTENT OF BODY RESERVES OF NUTRIENTS

NUTRIENT	TIME REQUIRED TO DEPLETE RESERVES IN WELL-NOURISHED INDIVIDUALS
Amino acids	Several hours
Carbohydrate	13 hours
Sodium	2-3 days
Water	4 days
Zinc	5 days
Fat	20-40 days
Thiamin	30-60 days
Vitamin C	60-120 days
Niacin	60-180 days
Riboflavin	60-180 days
Vitamin A	90-365 days
Iron	125 days (women), 750 days (men)
Iodine	1000 days
Calcium	2500 days

From Guthrie HA: *Introductory nutrition*, ed 7, St Louis, Mo., 1989, Mosby.

Page | 133

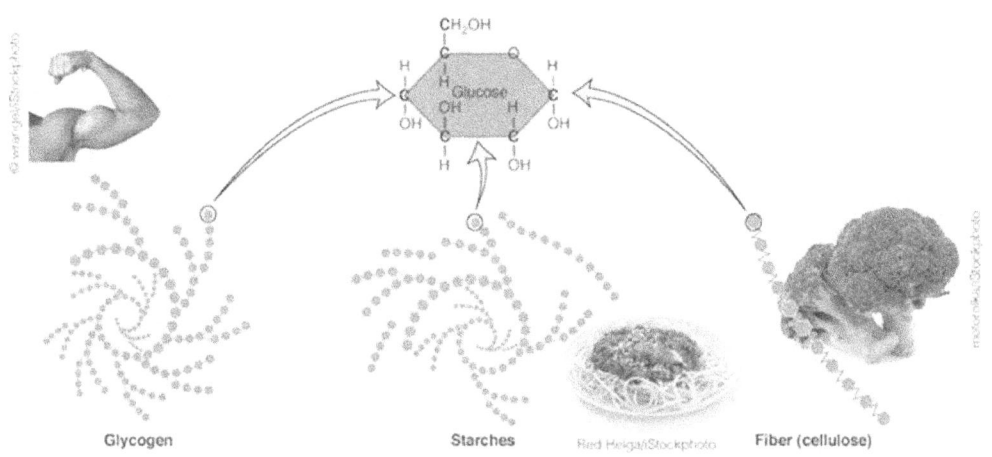

Glycogen

The polysaccharide glycogen is made of highly branched chains of glucose. This branched structure allows glycogen, which is found in muscle and liver, to be broken down quickly when the body needs glucose.

Starches

Different types of starch consist of either straight chains or branched chains of glucose. We consume a mixture of starches in grain products, legumes, and other starchy vegetables.

Fiber (cellulose)

Most fiber is made of either straight or branched chains of monosaccharides, but the bonds that link the sugar units cannot be broken by human digestive enzymes. For example, cellulose, shown here, is a fiber made up of straight chains of glucose molecules. Sources include wheat bran and broccoli.

The National Academy of Sciences' Institute of Medicine gives the following daily total fiber recommendations for adults

	Age 50 and younger	Age 51 and older
Men	38 grams	30 grams
Women	25 grams	21 grams

Foods with Soluble and Insoluble Fiber

Soluble Fiber	Insoluble Fiber

Soluble Fiber	Insoluble Fiber
• Apples	• Whole grain
• Pears	• Whole wheat breads
• Oranges	• Barley
• Peaches	• Brown rice
• Grapes	• Bulgur
• Prunes	• Whole-grain breakfast cereals
• Blueberries	• Wheat bran
• Strawberries	• Seeds
• Seeds and Nuts	• Vegetables:
• Oat bran	– Carrots
• Dried beans	– Cucumbers
• Oatmeal	– Zucchini
• Barley	– Celery
• Rye	– Tomatoes
• Vegetables	

Foods with High Fiber

Vegetables	Serving Size	Total fiber (grams)
Peas	1 cup	8.8
Potato, baked with skin	1 medium	4.4
Corn	1 cup	4.2
Popcorn, air-popped	3 cups	3.6
Tomato paste	¼ cup	3.0
Carrot	1 medium	2.0

Fruits	Serving Size	Total fiber (grams)
Apple, with skin	1 medium	4.4
Apricots, dried	10 halves	2.6
Raisins	1.5 ounce box	1.6
Orange	1 medium	3.1
Peaches, dried	3 halves	3.2
Blueberries	1 cup	3.5
Pear	1 medium	5.1

Understanding Carbohydrates: Life Energy, Fiber, Sugar & Starch!

Legumes, Nuts & Seeds	Serving Size	Total Fiber (grams)
Cashews	18 nuts	0.9
Peanuts	28 nuts	2.3
Pistachio nuts	47 nuts	2.9
Almonds	24 nuts	3.3
Baked beans, canned	1 cup	10.4
Lima beans	1 cup	13.2
Black beans	1 cup	15.0
Lentils	1 cup	15.6
Grains, Cereal & Pasta	Serving Size	Total Fiber (grams)
Bread, mixed grain	1 slice	1.7
Bread, whole-wheat	1 slice	1.9
Bread, rye	1 slice	1.9
Oatmeal	1 cup	4.0
Bran flakes	¾ cup	5.1
Spaghetti, whole-wheat	1 cup	6.3

Source: Adapted from the USDA National Nutrient Database for Standard Reference, Release 18. U.S. Department of Agriculture, Agricultural Research Service, 2005.

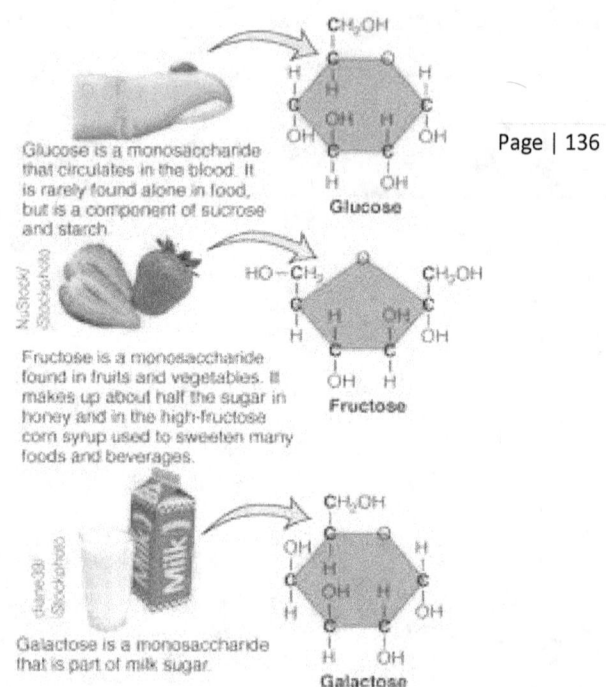

Glucose is a monosaccharide that circulates in the blood. It is rarely found alone in food, but is a component of sucrose and starch.

Glucose

Fructose is a monosaccharide found in fruits and vegetables. It makes up about half the sugar in honey and in the high-fructose corn syrup used to sweeten many foods and beverages.

Fructose

Galactose is a monosaccharide that is part of milk sugar.

Galactose

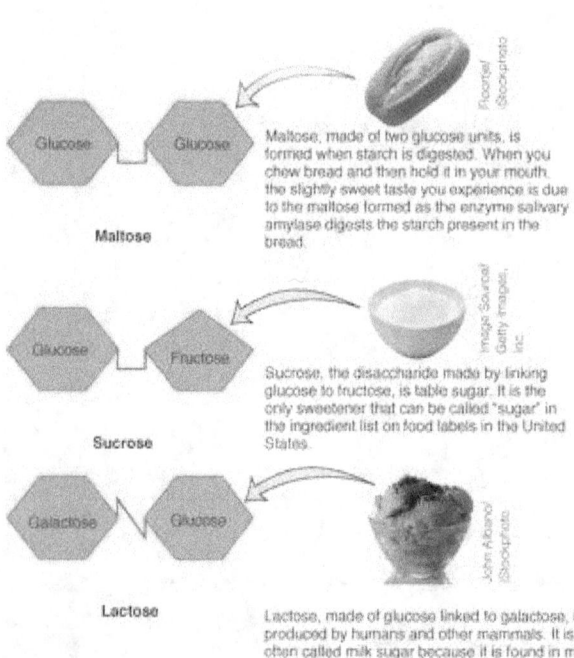

Maltose, made of two glucose units, is formed when starch is digested. When you chew bread and then hold it in your mouth, the slightly sweet taste you experience is due to the maltose formed as the enzyme salivary amylase digests the starch present in the bread.

Maltose

Sucrose, the disaccharide made by linking glucose to fructose, is table sugar. It is the only sweetener that can be called "sugar" in the ingredient list on food labels in the United States.

Sucrose

Lactose, made of glucose linked to galactose, is produced by humans and other mammals. It is often called milk sugar because it is found in milk, as well as ice cream, and other dairy products.

Lactose

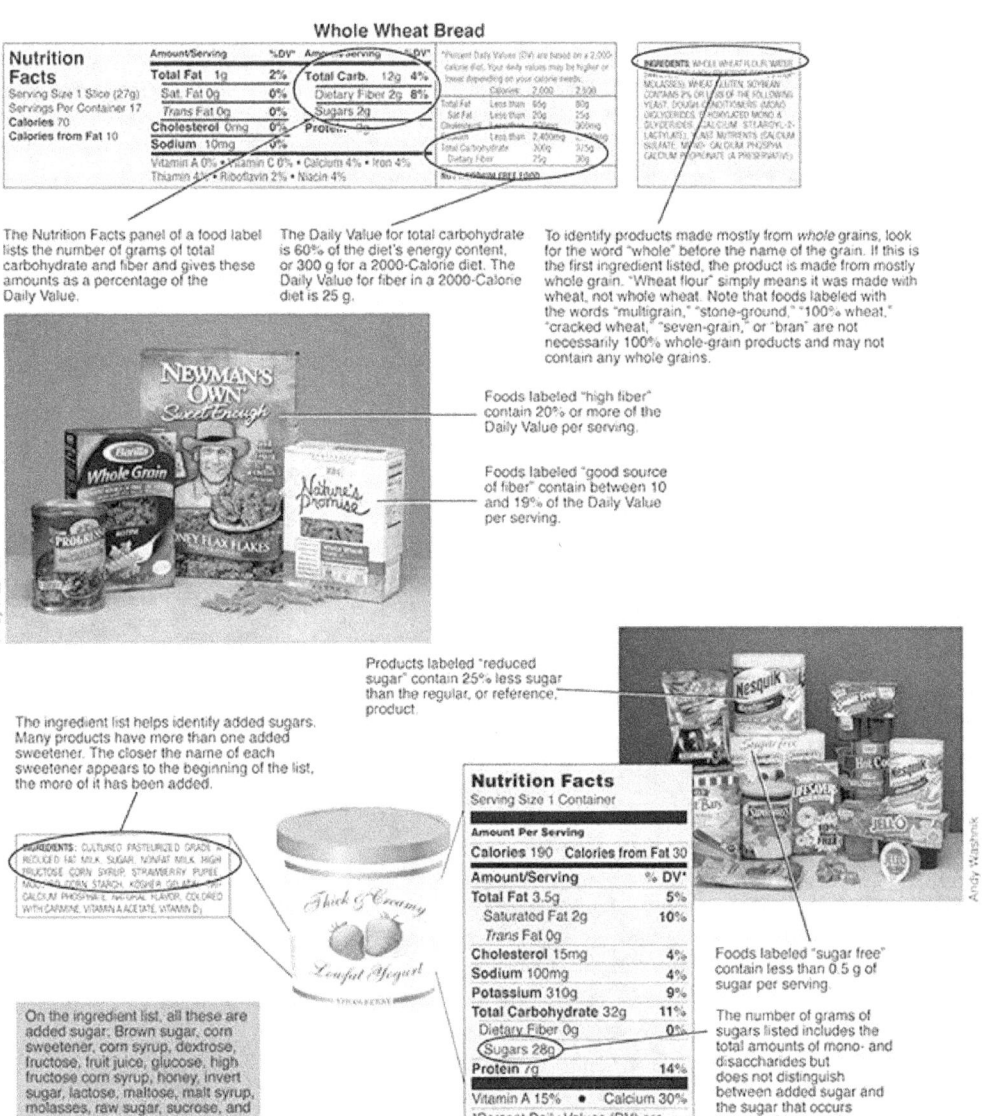

Whole Wheat Bread

The Nutrition Facts panel of a food label lists the number of grams of total carbohydrate and fiber and gives these amounts as a percentage of the Daily Value.

The Daily Value for total carbohydrate is 60% of the diet's energy content, or 300 g for a 2000-Calorie diet. The Daily Value for fiber in a 2000-Calorie diet is 25 g.

To identify products made mostly from *whole* grains, look for the word "whole" before the name of the grain. If this is the first ingredient listed, the product is made from mostly whole grain. "Wheat flour" simply means it was made with wheat, not whole wheat. Note that foods labeled with the words "multigrain," "stone-ground," "100% wheat," "cracked wheat," "seven-grain," or "bran" are not necessarily 100% whole-grain products and may not contain any whole grains.

Foods labeled "high fiber" contain 20% or more of the Daily Value per serving.

Foods labeled "good source of fiber" contain between 10 and 19% of the Daily Value per serving.

Products labeled "reduced sugar" contain 25% less sugar than the regular, or reference, product.

The ingredient list helps identify added sugars. Many products have more than one added sweetener. The closer the name of each sweetener appears to the beginning of the list, the more of it has been added.

On the ingredient list, all these are added sugar: Brown sugar, corn sweetener, corn syrup, dextrose, fructose, fruit juice, glucose, high fructose corn syrup, honey, invert sugar, lactose, maltose, malt syrup, molasses, raw sugar, sucrose, and sugar syrup concentrates.

Nutrition Facts

Serving Size 1 Container

Amount Per Serving	
Calories 190	Calories from Fat 30

Amount/Serving	% DV*
Total Fat 3.5g	5%
Saturated Fat 2g	10%
Trans Fat 0g	
Cholesterol 15mg	4%
Sodium 100mg	4%
Potassium 310mg	9%
Total Carbohydrate 32g	11%
Dietary Fiber 0g	0%
Sugars 28g	
Protein 7g	14%

Vitamin A 15% • Calcium 30%

*Percent Daily Values (DV) are based on a 2,000 calorie diet.

Foods labeled "sugar free" contain less than 0.5 g of sugar per serving.

The number of grams of sugars listed includes the total amounts of mono- and disaccharides but does not distinguish between added sugar and the sugar that occurs naturally in the food. Proposed changes to the Nutrition Facts include putting grams of added sugars as a separate line below Sugars.

① Glycolysis, which takes place in the cytosol, splits glucose, a six-carbon molecule, into two three-carbon molecules (pyruvate). This step releases high-energy electrons (purple balls) and produces a small amount of ATP. Pyruvate is then either broken down to produce more ATP or is used to remake glucose.

② Pyruvate can be used to produce more ATP when oxygen is available. In the mitochondria, pyruvate is broken down, releasing carbon dioxide (CO_2) and high-energy electrons and forming acetyl-CoA (2 carbons), which continues through aerobic metabolism.

③ Acetyl-CoA enters the citric acid cycle, where carbon dioxide and high-energy electrons are released and where a small amount of ATP is produced.

④ Most ATP is produced in the final step of aerobic metabolism. Here the energy in the high-energy electrons released in previous steps is transferred to ATP, and the electrons are combined with oxygen and hydrogen to form water.

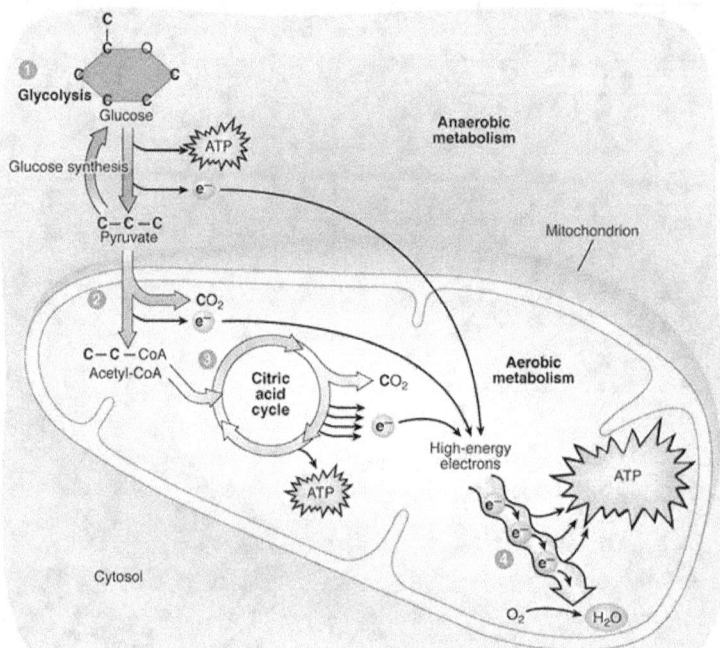

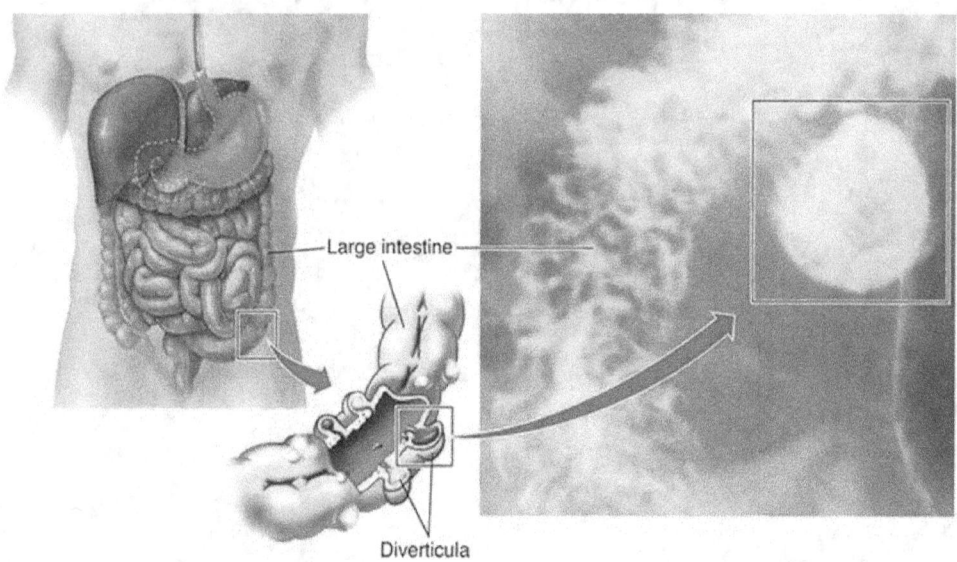

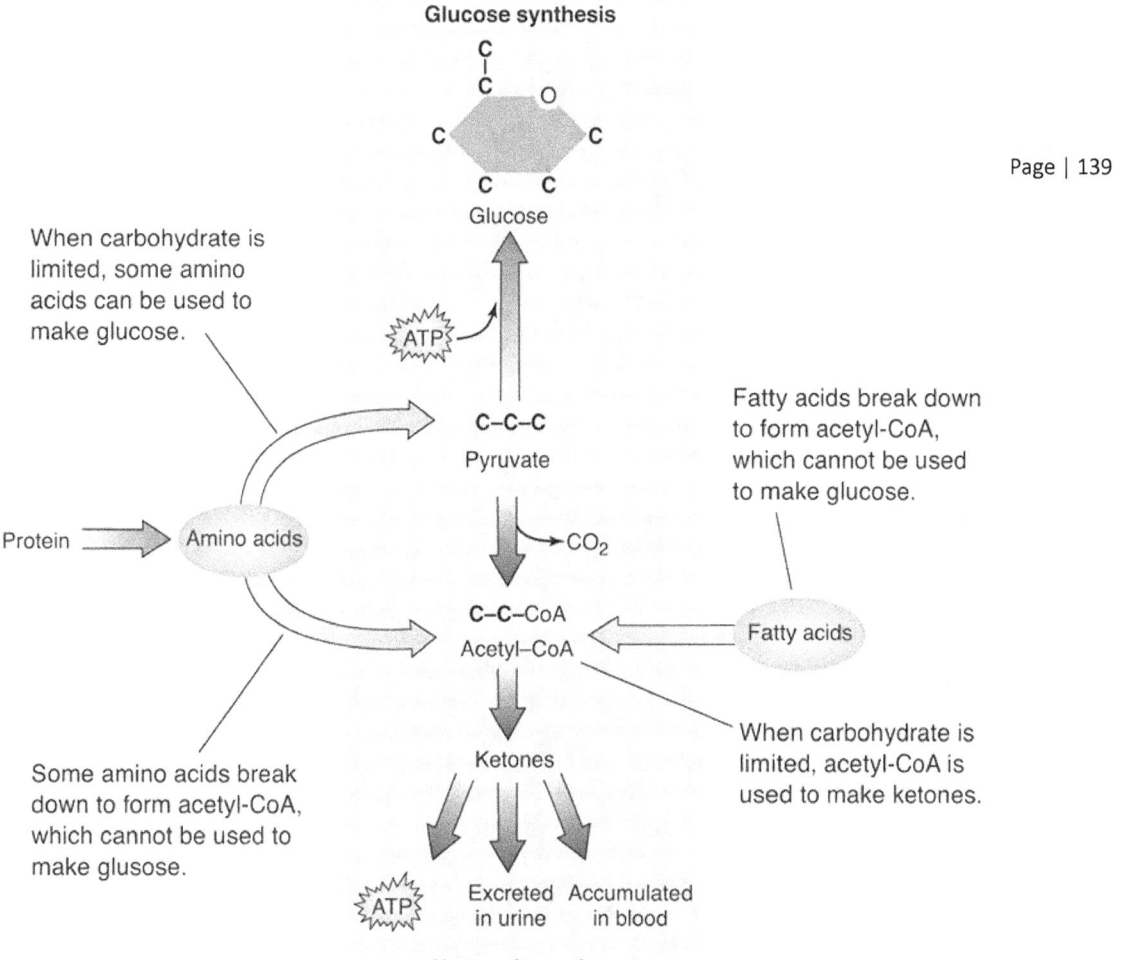

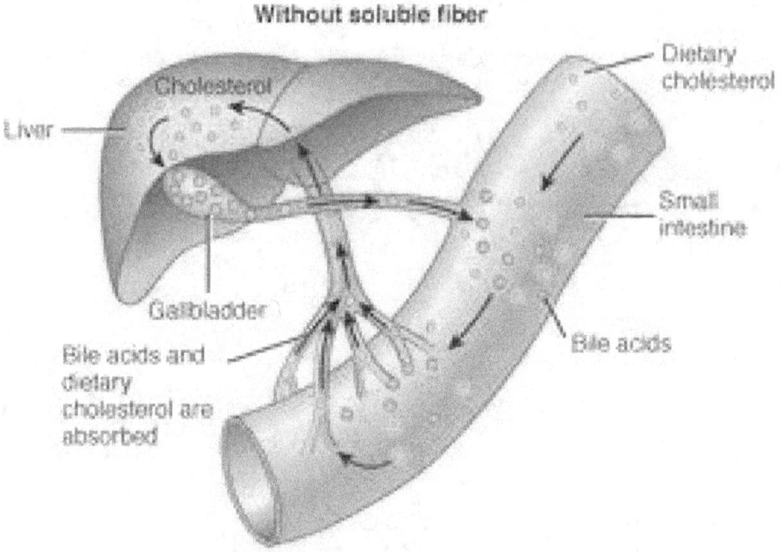

Without soluble fiber

Cholesterol

Dietary cholesterol

Liver

Small intestine

Gallbladder

Bile acids and dietary cholesterol are absorbed

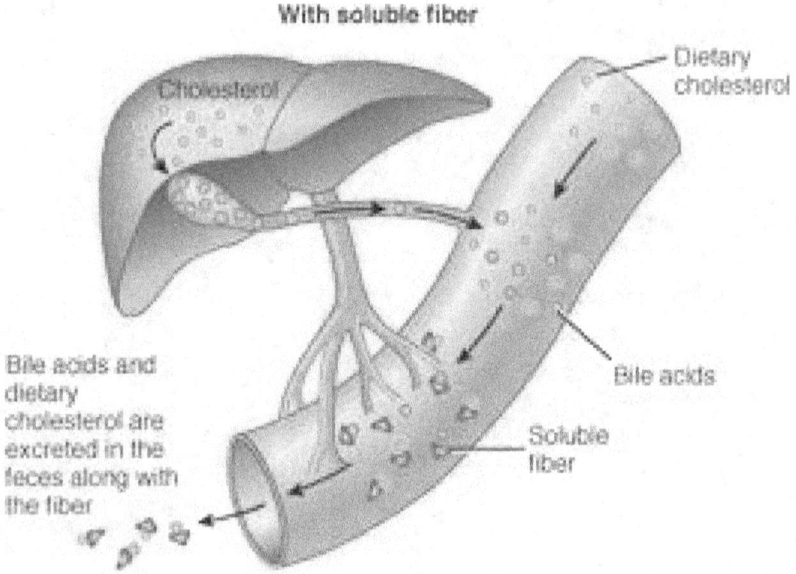

Bile acids

With soluble fiber

Dietary cholesterol

Cholesterol

Bile acids

Bile acids and dietary cholesterol are excreted in the feces along with the fiber

Soluble fiber

Key Terms

* * * * *

Carbohydrate Compound made up of carbon, hydrogen, and oxygen; includes starches, sugars, and dietary fiber made and stored in plants; digestible carbohydrates yield 4 kcal/g.

Dextrin: Intermediate breakdown product in the digestion of Starch.

Cariogenic: Promotes the development of dental caries or tooth decay.

Dietary fiber: Nondigestible Carbohydrates and Lignin found in Plants; dietary fiber is eaten as an intact part of the plant in which it is found.

Disaccharides: Class of sugars composed of two molecules of monosaccharide. The three most common disaccharides are sucrose, lactose, and maltose high-density lipoprotein (HDL) cholesterol A lipoprotein produced in the liver that carries cholesterol from the tissues back to the liver for degradation and elimination.

Glycogen: A polysaccharide made up of many saccharide (glucose) units. Glycogen is the body storage form of carbohydrate (glucose) found mostly in the liver, with lesser amounts in the muscle.

Low-Density Lipoprotein (LDL) Cholesterol: A lipoprotein produced in the liver that transports fatty acids and cholesterol to the cells and tissues; this lipoprotein contains a high proportion of cholesterol.

Metabolism: Sum of all the various biochemical and physiologic processes by which the body grows and maintains itself (anabolism), breaks down and reshapes tissue (catabolism), and transforms energy to do its work. Products of these various reactions are called *metabolites.*

Monosaccharide: Simple sugar; a carbohydrate containing a single saccharide (sugar) unit. The most common monosaccharides are glucose, galactose, and fructose.

Oligosaccharides: Intermediate products of polysaccharide digestion that contain from 3 to 10 glucose units.

Nonnutritive sweeteners: TOXIC Substances with sweetening power that are not efficiently absorbed or cannot be metabolized to provide energy or can be used in very minute amounts based on their intense sweetness.

Photosynthesis: Process by which plants containing chlorophyll are able to manufacture carbohydrate by combining CO_2 from the air and water from the soil with sunlight providing energy and chlorophyll as a catalyst.

Sugar Alcohols: Alcohol formed from a simple sugar; sugar alcohols do not react with bacteria in the mouth to form dental caries; most sugar alcohols are poorly digested and absorbed, and yield less than 4 kcal/g.

Understanding Carbohydrates: Life Energy, Fiber, Sugar & Starch!

Functional Fiber: Non-digestible Carbohydrates isolated from plant foods or synthesized and added to foods to increase their fiber content.

Total Fiber Dietary: Fiber plus functional Fiber; the total amount of fiber in an individual's diet from all sources.

Energy Density: The relative number of kcalories per unit weight of food; foods high in fat and added sugar have high energy density; vegetables that contain large amounts of water and fiber have low energy density.

Amylase: A digestive enzyme that breaks down starch; salivary amylase begins the digestion of starch in the mouth; pancreatic amylase enters the small intestine as part of the pancreatic secretions to continue starch breakdown in the duodenum.

Sucrose: Enzyme that splits the disaccharide sucrose, releasing the monosaccharides glucose and fructose.

Lactase: Enzyme that splits the disaccharide lactose, releasing the monosaccharides glucose and galactose.

Maltase: Enzyme that splits the disaccharide maltose, releasing two units of the monosaccharide glucose.

Portal: An entryway, usually referring to the portal circulation of blood that delivers nutrients absorbed from the small intestine to the liver.

- acceptable daily intake
- aerobic metabolism
- anaerobic metabolism
- autoimmune disease
- bran
- cellulose
- complex carbohydrate
- diabetes mellitus
- disaccharide
- diverticula
- diverticulitis
- diverticulosis
- endosperm

- enrichment

- fasting hypoglycemia

- fiber

- fructose

- galactose

- germ

- gestational diabetes

- glucagon

- glucose

- glycemic index

- glycemic load

- glycemic response

- glycogen

- glycolysis

- hemorrhoid

- hypoglycemia

- insoluble fiber

- insulin

- insulin resistance

- ketoacidosis

- ketone or ketone body

- ketosis

- lactose

- lactose intolerance

- maltose

- monosaccharide

- nonnutritive sweetener or artificial sweetener

- oligosaccharide

- photosynthesis
- polysaccharide
- prediabetes
- reactive hypoglycemia
- refined
- resistant starch
- simple carbohydrate
- soluble fiber
- starch
- sucrose
- sugar unit
- type 1 diabetes
- type 2 diabetes
- unrefined food
- whole-grain product

Howley, Edward. *Fitness Professional's Handbook, 6th Edition.* Human Kinetics, 04/2012.

Mahan LK, Escott-Stump S: *Krause's food and nutrition therapy,* ed 12, St Louis, Mo., 2008, Saunders.)

Thygerson, Alton L. *Fit to Be Well: Essential Concepts, 3rd Edition.* Jones & Bartlett Learning, 20120213. VitalBook file.

The National Digestive Diseases Information Clearinghouse (NDDIC), National Institute of Diabetes and Digestive and Kidney Diseases (NIDDK), and National Institutes of Health of the U.S. Department of Health and Human Services. Lactose intolerance. Available online at http://digestive.niddk.nih.gov/ddiseases/pubs/lactoseintolerance/. Accessed May 13, 2014.

Kumar, V., Sinha, A.K., Makkar, H.P., et al. Dietary roles of non-starch polysaccharides in human nutrition: A review. *Crit Rev Food Sci Nutr 52*:899-935, 2012.

American Diabetes Association. Standards of medical care in diabetes—2014. *Diabetes Care* 37:S14-S80, 2014

Salas-Salvadó, J., Martinez-González, M.Á., Bulló, M., and Ros, E. The role of diet in the prevention of type 2 diabetes. *Nutr Metab Cardiovasc Dis 21*(Suppl 2):B32-B48, 2011.

Silva, F.M., Kramer, C.K., de Almeida J.C., et al. Fiber intake and glycemic control in patients with type 2 diabetes mellitus: A systematic review with meta-analysis of randomized controlled trials. *Nutr Rev 71*:790-801, 2013.

InterAct consortium. Consumption of sweet beverages and type 2 diabetes incidence in European adults: Results from EPICInterAct. *Diabetologia 56*:1520-1530, 2013.

Rippe, J.M., and Angelopoulos, T.J. Sucrose, high-fructose corn syrup, and fructose, their metabolism and potential health effects: What do we really know? *Adv Nutr 4*:236-245, 2013.

Johnson, R.K., Appel, L.J., Brands, M., et al. Dietary sugars intake and cardiovascular health: A scientific statement from the American Heart Association on behalf of the American Heart Association Nutrition Committee of the Council on Nutrition, Physical Activity, and Metabolism and the Council on Epidemiology and Prevention. Circulation *120*:1011-1020, 2009.

Centers for Disease Control and Prevention. National diabetes fact sheet: national estimates and general information on diabetes and prediabetes in the United States, 2011. Atlanta, GA: U.S. Department of Health and Human Services, Centers for Disease Control and Prevention, 2011

The Food and Nutrition Board of the Institute of Medicine has established *Dietary Reference Intakes* (DRIs) to help people achieve a healthy intake of nutrients and some of the data is used here to support the premise that Carbohydrates are an essential, if not the ONE essential element to our Health and Wellness. The *DRIs* consist of the recommended intakes of Nutrients based on the two uncontrollable aspects - Age and Sex. There are four main categories that form the foundation of the DRIs, which include: *Recommended Dietary Allowances* (RDAs), which are the amounts found to be adequate for approximately 97% of the population. *Adequate Intakes* (AIs), which are the amounts considered adequate although insufficient data exist to establish the appropriate RDA. *Tolerable Upper Intake Levels* (UL), which are the highest intakes believed to pose no health risk. *Acceptable Macronutrient Distribution Ranges* (AMDRs) have been established for Fats, Carbohydrates, and Proteins. The reports from the Institute of Medicine can be retrieved at the *National Academies Press* website (www.nap.edu).

More Titles Published By Supreme Health and Fitness!

OxyGen: The Breath Of LIFE In Atomic Form
Authored by Sean Ali

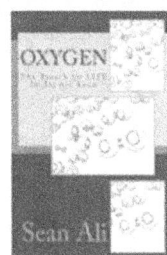

List Price: **$30.00**

6" x 9" (15.24 x 22.86 cm)
Full Color on White paper
134 pages

ISBN-13: 978-1541272170 (CreateSpace-Assigned)
ISBN-10: 154127217X
BISAC: Health & Fitness / Healthy Living

Peace and Blessings of Health!

"Do YOU have health issues that YOU want to over-come?
"Do YOU want to Improve the Quality of YOUR Life?
"Do YOU want to achieve ABUNDANT LIFE?
*** THEN THIS BOOK IS FOR YOU!! ***

Oxygen IS the Breath Of LIFE in Atomic form!

This short work is a composition of Scientific, Medical and Spiritually based research , compiled into a comprehensive, easily read and understood format, designed to Help the reader achieve and maintain their own Supreme Health and Fitness!

We have 3 major functions - Eating, Drinking and Breathing, that must be performed in order for us to be considered Alive .... Of these 3 functions, Breathing is the least explored, taught or performed properly - BUT THE MOST IMPORTANT

We can go 7-10 days without Food before signs of Nutritional deficiency. We can go 3-7 days without Water before we present symptoms...... But, 1 Minute of Oxygen deprivation/deficiency causes Cellular Damage!

Our Cells need 2 elements for Growth and Reproduction = OXYGEN & GLUCOSE !

Let's explore and discover the Amazing Power of Oxygen and the Natural Ability to Heal Self!

OXYGEN IS THE BREATH OF LIFE IN ATOMIC FORM !

OPEN THIS BOOK - and take the steps to Successfully Build Your own Supreme Health & Fitness!

PEACE!

LIFE Energy: The Sun, Glucose & WHY Humans Are Herbivores!
Authored by Sean Ali

List Price: **$30.00**

6" x 9" (15.24 x 22.86 cm)
Full Color on White paper
156 pages

ISBN-13: 978-1544622842 (CreateSpace-Assigned)
ISBN-10: 1544622848
BISAC: Medical / Diet Therapy

Peace and Blessings of Health!

*Do YOU have a health issue that YOU would like to over-come?
*Do YOU want to Improve the Quality of YOUR Life?
*Do YOU want to experience ABUNDANT LIFE?

*** OPEN THIS BOOK - NOW!!! ***

This small book is written with the purpose of re-examining the role of Nutrition in health care and everyday Life......LIFE IS ENERGY.....Nutrition is a descriptive term to describe how we replenish our Life Energy.
Understanding Nutrition is the equivalent of understanding Energy
Knowledge of Nutrition enables us to make precise Energy adjustments through Nutrients to provide the proper Energy needed for all our body functions/tasks – from achieving Homeostasis, facilitating our Growth, Development and Self-Healing.
We come from the Earth and all our Solutions are manifested from the Earth...... All we have to do is return back to the Earth and extract what we need.
Food is our naturally occurring vehicle, perfectly designed for administering the Life Energy in the form of Nutrition.
Our Food choices and the Energy released from it, presents as either the root cause of our dis-ease or the base for our Solution.
From our Cells to our Immune system, we are Created to Heal and Regenerate Self with the aide of proper Nutrition/Energy.
Our Food is our Medicine ONLY with proper application...... There is no in-between, which means that we are either eating to die – OR – Eating To LIVE !!!!
Energy is the Key to LIFE and we Know that the Sun is the Source of all Energy, so if we focus on how to obtain as much Sun in the form of food as possible = the Key to Nutritional Health and Therapy.
Let us explore and examine Life Energy and how to obtain the best Quality and Value so that we may successfully manifest the Best out of Life and Enjoy a long, active and fruitful Life-span!

Achieving and Maintaining Supreme Health and Fitness by increasing the level of Knowledge and Science of Life!

Peace
Sean Ali

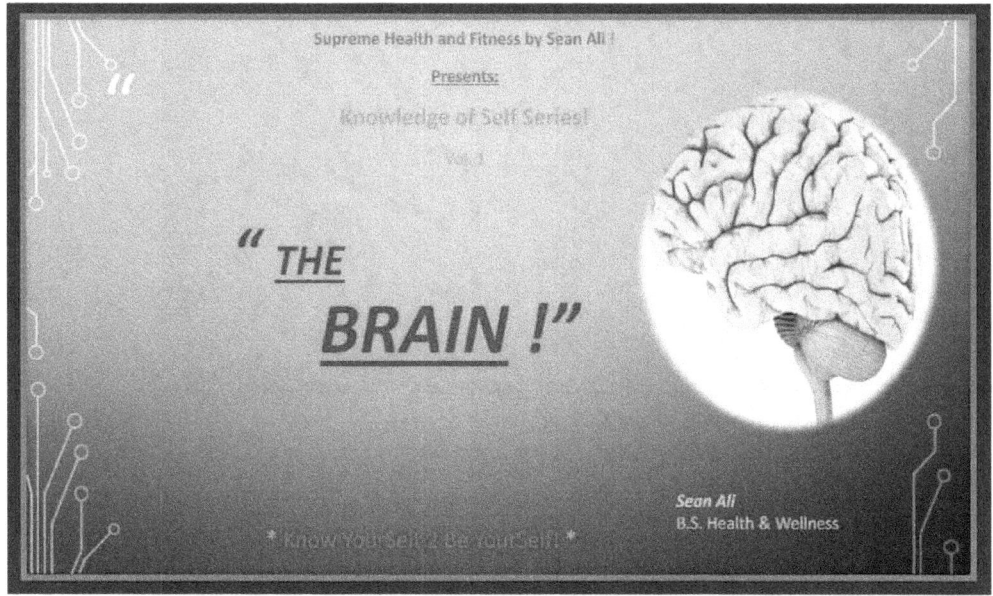

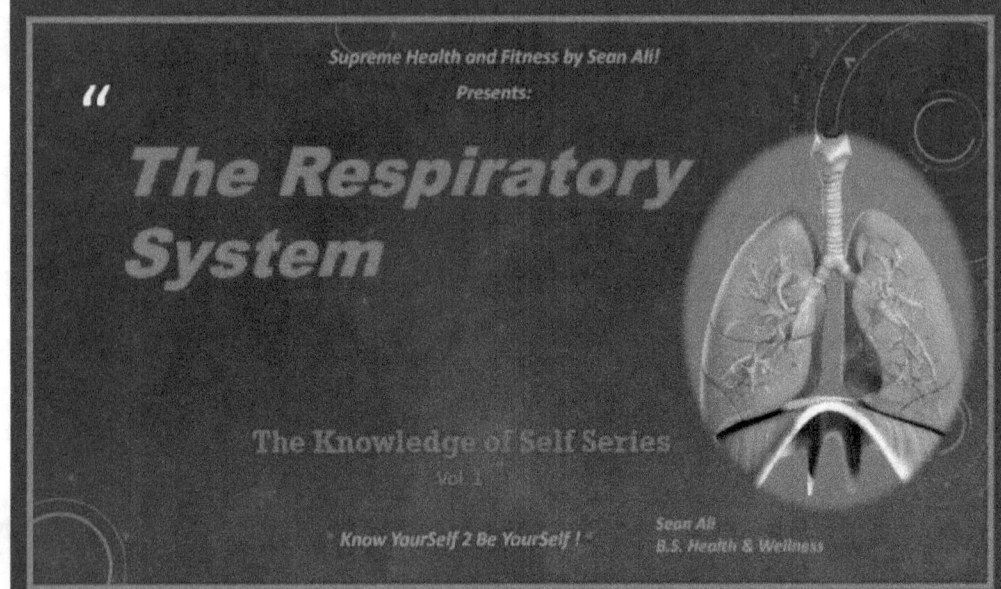

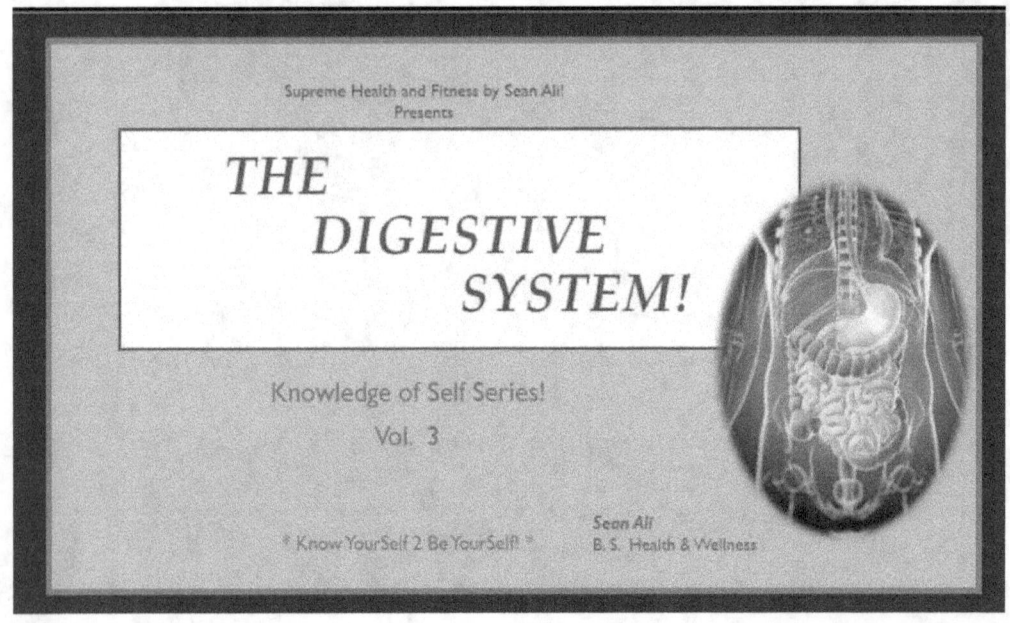

Abundant Life Series!

Project Summary

Enjoying Abundant LIFE!: Scientific Concepts to Successfully Build YOUR Supreme Health!

Authored by Sean Ali

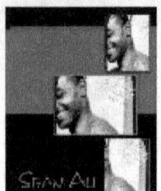

List Price: **$35.00**

8" x 10" (20.32 x 25.4 cm)
Full Color on White paper
170 pages

ISBN-13: 978-1546732075 (CreateSpace-Assigned)
ISBN-10: 1546732071
BISAC: Medical / Healing

Peace and Blessings of Health!

*Do YOU have a health issue that YOU would like to over-come?
*Do YOU want to improve the Quality of YOUR Life?
*Do YOU want to experience ABUNDANT LIFE?

*** OPEN THIS BOOK - NOW!!! ***

This small book is written with the purpose of re-examining the role of Nutrition in health care and everyday Life......LIFE IS ENERGY.....Nutrition is a descriptive term to describe how we replenish our Life Energy.

Understanding Nutrition is the equivalent of understanding Energy

Knowledge of Nutrition enables us to make precise Energy adjustments through Nutrients to provide the proper Energy needed for all our body functions/tasks -- from achieving Homeostasis, facilitating our Growth, Development and Self-Healing.

We come from the Earth and all our Solutions are manifested from the Earth...... All we have to do is return back to the Earth and extract what we need.

Food is our naturally occurring vehicle, perfectly designed for administering the Life Energy in the form of Nutrition.

Our Food choices and the Energy released from it, presents as either the root cause of our dis-ease or the base for our Solution.

From our Cells to our Immune system, we are Created to Heal and Regenerate Self with the aide of proper Nutrition/Energy.

Our Food is our Medicine ONLY with proper application...... There is no in-between, which means that we are either eating to die - OR - Eating To LIVE !!!!

Energy is the Key to LIFE and we Know that the Sun is the Source of all Energy, so if we focus on how to obtain as much Sun in the form of food as possible = the Key to Nutritional Health and Therapy.

Let us explore and examine Life Energy and how to obtain the best Quality and Value so that we may successfully manifest the Best out of Life and Enjoy a long, active and fruitful Life-span!

Achieving and Maintaining Supreme Health and Fitness by increasing the level of Knowledge and Science of Life!

Peace
Sean Ali

CreateSpace eStore: https://www.createspace.com/7174743

Project Summary

Understanding Our Human Energy!: Energy Cycle & Transformation to Achieve Abundant LIFE!

Authored by Sean Ali

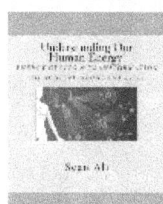

List Price: **$45.00**

8" x 10" (20.32 x 25.4 cm)
Full Color on White paper
224 pages

ISBN-13: 978-1546343462 (CreateSpace-Assigned)
ISBN-10: 1546343466
BISAC: Medical / Alternative Medicine

Peace and Blessings of Life!

·Do YOU Have health ailments/issues that YOU would like to over-come??
·Do YOU want to Improve the Quality of YOUR Life??
·Do YOU want to Experience and Enjoy ABUNDANT LIFE??
** Then this book is for YOU!

This small book is written so that we can explore and gain an Understanding of what our Human Energy System is, with a particular focus on What our Energy is, the Best sources and What to avoid to successfully Grow and LIVE so that we can Enjoy to the fullest, our GOD-Given potential of a Long and Abundant LIFE !!!!!!
Understanding our Human Energy is synonymous with Understanding our LIFE...it's what keeps us Alive and the main difference between Us and a body in the grave - Human Energy !!!!
Human Energy is manifested in the form of FOOD... Growing Our Own Food is the ONLY way that ensures we recieve the Highest Quality Life Energy - Straight from the Source!

OPEN THIS BOOK and Begin the neccessary steps to Improve the Quality of YOUR LIFE!

Building and Maintaining Supreme Health & Fitness by increasing the level of Knowledge and Science of Life!

Peace!
Sean Ali, BS Health & Wellness

CreateSpace eStore: https://www.createspace.com/7126564

Science Of Healing Series!

Project Summary

The Manual Of Healing Herbal Elements!: *Earth-based Solutions for Healing, Health & Life!*
Authored by Sean Ali, Authored by Kareem Tyree, Authored by Gabriella Monique, Authored by Khalil Malik

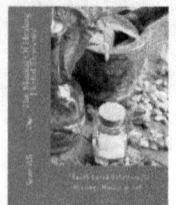

List Price: **$65.00**

8" x 10" (20.32 x 25.4 cm)
Full Color on White paper
336 pages

ISBN-13: **978-1547137985** (CreateSpace-Assigned)
ISBN-10: **1547137983**
BISAC: Medical / Holistic Medicine

Peace and Blessings of Health!
This small work is being presented as a Manual of Healing, Health and Life. A comprehensive and scientific Handbook of Analysis and Research on over 80 Clinically & Commonly accessible Life & Healing Energy Herbal Elements. Each Herbal Element is categorized to include the latest research on the Uses, Actions, Dosages, Client Considerations, Contraindications & Interactions.
As many of Us are witnessing the RISE in Life-threatening dis-eases, especially in childhood Obesity and Diabetes, we are looking for more Natural ways to Heal.
This Manual Of Healing is a Professional Grade handbook to Help YOU choose and use the BEST Naturally occurring Life Elements to Successfully Heal YourSelf!
We come from the Earth and ALL our Solutions come from the Earth!

PEACE!
Sean Ali

CreateSpace eStore: https://www.createspace.com/7225520

Project Summary
Understanding & Creating Herbal Healing!: Teas, Decoctions & Tinctures!
Authored by Sean Ali, Authored by Khalil Malik, Authored by Kareem Tyree, Authored by Gabriella Monique

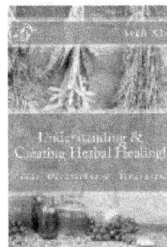

List Price: **$22.00**

7" x 10" (17.78 x 25.4 cm)
Full Color on White paper
108 pages

ISBN-13: **978-1548105457** (CreateSpace-Assigned)
ISBN-10: **1548105457**
BISAC: Medical / Healing

Peace and Blessings of Health!

This small work represents Volume 2 of my Science Of Healing Series and is being presented as a Handbook of Healing through the vehicles of Teas, Decoctions and Tinctures.

This is a comprehensive and scientific Handbook of Analysis and Research on over 30 Clinically used & easily accessible Life & Healing Energy Herbal Elements.

This Handbook Of Healing is Professional Grade and designed specifically to Help YOU choose and use the BEST Naturally occurring Life Elements to Successfully Heal YourSelf!
We come from the Earth and ALL our Solutions come from the Earth!

PEACE!
Sean Ali

CreateSpace eStore: https://www.createspace.com/7257513

Sean Ali

Understanding Carbohydrates: LIFE Energy, Fiber, Sugar and Starch! (Science Of LIFE Series)

ISBN-13: 978-1520559988, **ISBN-10:** 1520559984

#1 New Release in Fiber

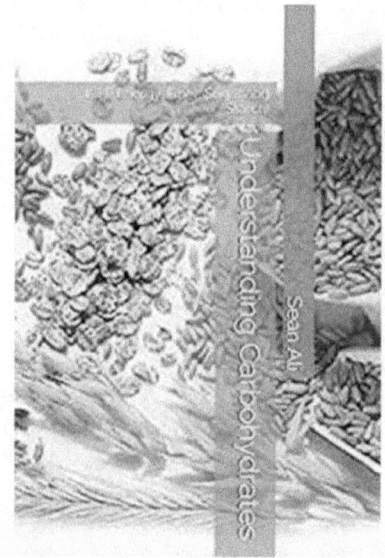

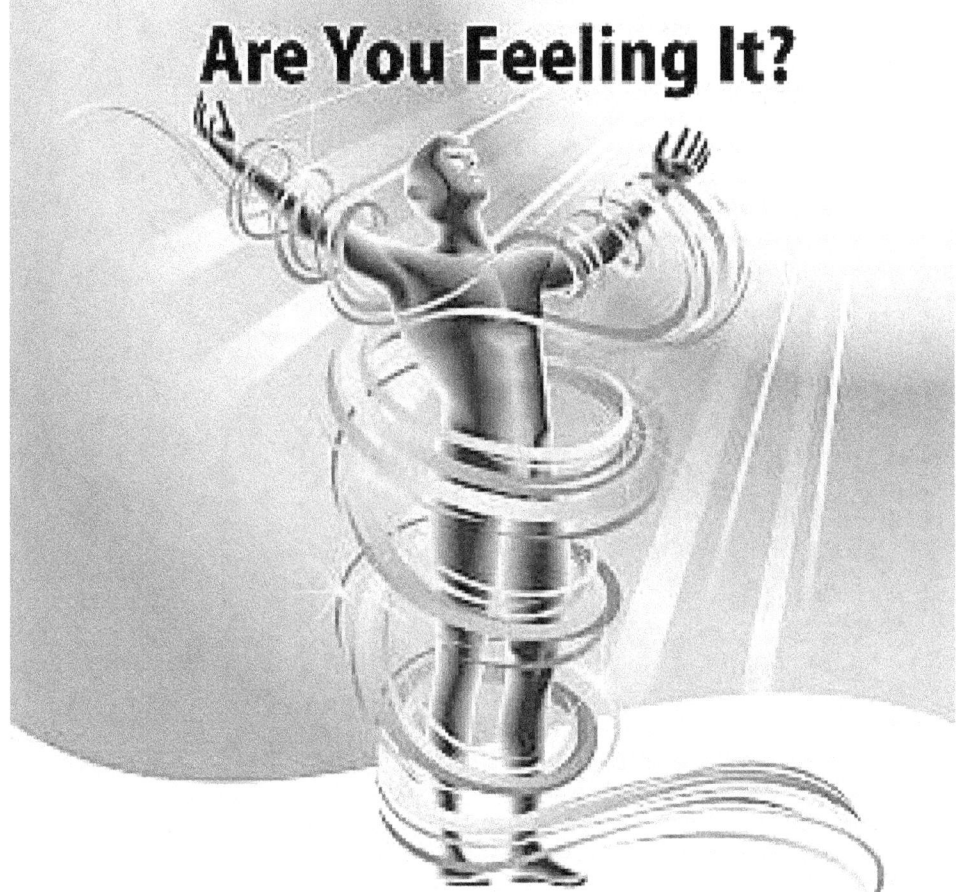